THE DIARY OF
SIR DAVID HAMILTON
1709–1714

THE DIARY OF
Sir David Hamilton
1709–1714

EDITED BY

PHILIP ROBERTS

OXFORD
AT THE CLARENDON PRESS
1975

Oxford University Press, Ely House, London W. I

GLASGOW NEW YORK TORONTO MELBOURNE WELLINGTON
CAPE TOWN IBADAN NAIROBI DAR ES SALAAM LUSAKA ADDIS ABABA
DELHI BOMBAY CALCUTTA MADRAS KARACHI LAHORE DACCA
KUALA LUMPUR SINGAPORE HONG KONG TOKYO

ISBN 0 19 822364 1

Printed in Great Britain
at the University Press, Oxford
by Vivian Ridler
Printer to the University

FOR KATE

PREFACE

It is appropriate that I record separately my obligation to my colleague, Dr. W. A. Speck of the Department of History, University of Newcastle upon Tyne, who has supplied the historical annotations to this book. I have drawn freely on his time and generosity in preparing the diary for publication. Without his advice and knowledge this work would have been the poorer.

ACKNOWLEDGEMENTS

MY thanks are owing to the following people and institutions: Lady Monica Salmond and Peter Walne, Esq., County Archivist of Hertfordshire, for permission to publish the diary; the staff of Hertfordshire R.O. for their help in making freely available the Panshanger Manuscripts; the Duke of Marlborough for allowing me access to the Blenheim archive; the Director of Public Libraries and his colleagues at Motherwell, where the Hamilton of Dalzell papers are presently stored; the librarian of the Royal College of Physicians, London, whose patience and courtesy is endless; Miss J. S. Emmerson, Keeper of the Pybus Collection, University of Newcastle upon Tyne; the librarian, the Royal Society of Medicine; the Keeper of Manuscripts, University of Edinburgh; the Curator of Historical Records, the Scottish Record Office; the librarian, the Wellcome Institute of the History of Medicine; the librarian of the Beinecke Rare Books Library, University of Yale; Mrs. Marion S. Pottle, Cataloguer of the Boswell Papers at Yale University; William Heinemann Ltd.; K. Monkman, Esq.; the County Archivist, Wiltshire; the staff of the British Museum, the Bodleian Library, the Public Record Office, and the Guildhall Library.

I am most grateful to Professor Geoffrey Holmes for his generous advice and Dr. R. K. R. Thornton for reading the typescript and making valuable suggestions which I have tried to incorporate.

The Research Committee of the University of Newcastle upon Tyne gave financial assistance towards the cost of producing this work, and the University Court granted me a term's leave of absence in order to complete the final version.

P. R.

Newcastle upon Tyne

CONTENTS

ABBREVIATIONS xiii

NOTE ON DATES xv

INTRODUCTION xvii
1. A Biographical Sketch of David Hamilton xix
2. Hamilton's Medical Theories and his Practice xxv
3. Hamilton in Politics: Whig, Royal Confidant, and Political Broker xxxi

NOTE ON THE TEXT xlvii

THE DIARY 1

NOTES 70

APPENDICES
A. The Queen and the Duchess, 1–18 January 1711 107
B. Hamilton's Scottish Circle 111
C. The Contents List of the Original Diary 115
D. Godolphin's Advice to the Queen 127

BIBLIOGRAPHY 128

INDEX 135

ABBREVIATIONS

Add. MSS.	British Museum, Additional MSS.
Blenheim MSS.	MSS. of His Grace the Duke of Marlborough, Blenheim Palace, Woodstock
Boswell Papers	Papers of James Boswell, Beinecke Rare Books Library, University of Yale. (i) Talbot Papers, Inventory no. 2, Hamilton to James Boswell. (ii) Ibid., Inventory no. 6, Lady Overkirk to Elizabeth Boswell
BM	British Museum
Bod.	Bodleian Library, Oxford
Bolingbroke, *Correspondence*	*Letters and Correspondence . . . of Henry St. John, Lord Viscount Bolingbroke* ed. G. Parke (1798)
Boyer, *Annals*	A. Boyer, *History of the Reign of Queen Anne digested into Annals* (1703–13)
Boyer, *Political State*	A. Boyer, *The Political State of Great Britain* (1718)
Burnet	*Bishop Burnet's History of His Own Time* (Oxford, 1833)
Cal. Treas. Bks.	*Calendar of Treasury Books*
Cal. Treas. Papers	*Calendar of Treasury Papers*
Cal. S.P. Dom.	*Calendar of State Papers, Domestic Series*
Cobbett, *Parliamentary History*	W. Cobbett, *The Parliamentary History of England* (1806–12)
Commons Journal	*House of Commons Journals*
Conduct	*An Account of the Conduct of the Duchess of Marlborough* (1742)
Cowper, *Diary*	*The Private Diary of William, First Earl Cowper*, ed. E. C. Hawtry (Roxburgh Club, 1833)
Coxe	*Memoirs of the Duke of Marlborough*, by Archdeacon Coxe, new. edn. rev. by J. Wade, (1905–8)
DNB	*Dictionary of National Biography*
Foster	Foster, J., *Alumni Oxonienses 1500–1714* (1891–2); *Alumni Oxonienses 1715–1886* (1887–8)
Green, *Sarah*	David Green, *Sarah Duchess of Marlborough* (1967)
HMC	Historical Manuscripts Commission
Holmes	Geoffrey Holmes, *British Politics in the Age of Anne* (1967)

ABBREVIATIONS

Holmes, *Trial*	Geoffrey Holmes, *The Trial of Doctor Sacheverell* (1973)
Luttrell	Narcissus Luttrell, *A Brief Historical Relation of State Affairs* . . . (Oxford, 1857)
Mary Cowper, Diary	The Diary of Mary, Countess Cowper, Panshanger MSS., D/EP F. 205, Hertford Record Office
Orbiston Letters	MS. letters to the family of Hamilton of Orbiston and Dalzell, Motherwell Public Library
Panshanger MSS.	Panshanger MSS., Hertford Record Office
Priv. Corr.	*Private Correspondence of Sarah, Duchess of Marlborough* (1838)
PRO	Public Record Office
PRO, L.C.	Public Record Office, Lord Chamberlain's Papers
RO	County Record Office
Royal College of Physicians, 'Annals'	MSS. Annals (Contemporary Transcript, vols. v–viii, 1682–1722)
Strickland	Strickland, Agnes, *Lives of the Queens of England* (1851, 2)
Swift, *Journal*	*Journal to Stella*, ed. H. Williams, (1948)
Wentworth Papers	*The Wentworth Papers 1705–1739* (ed. J. J. Cartwright, 1883)

NOTE ON DATES

ALL dates are given in the Old Style of the Julian Calendar, but it is assumed that each new year begins on 1 January. Occasional references to documents written from the Continent or by Continental envoys or agents in London are dated by both their Old and New Style dates.

INTRODUCTION

HAMILTON, DAVID (1663–1721): born Lanarkshire, the youngest son of the first Laird of Dalzell, matriculated at the University of Leyden 1683, M.D. Rheims 1686; Licentiate of the College of Physicians 1688; married first wife 1689, second wife 1694. Thomas born 1695, David in 1700; Knighted and elected Fellow of the College of Physicians 1703; appointed third physician-in-ordinary to Queen Anne 1703; F.R.S. 1708; called to attend on the Queen at the end of 1708; 1712 appointed second physician to the Queen; parted from his wife 1713; appointed physician to Princess of Wales 1714; died August 1721 and was buried in St. Katherine Coleman, Fenchurch Street.

SIR DAVID HAMILTON'S record of his attendance as a physician-in-ordinary upon Queen Anne provides a unique account through his eyes of many of the events, crises, and developments of the last four years of the Queen's reign. From December 1709 until Anne's death he recorded, sometimes briefly, sometimes in great detail, the Queen's ideas and opinions, the reactions of some of her ministers, and the mood of the times. What he presents amounts to an intimate portrait of Queen Anne and a valuable version of one of the most complex periods in English history.

On 18 March 1715 Hamilton sent to his friend, Mary, Countess Cowper, wife of the Lord Chancellor in the first Whig administration of George I, 'a Copy of a great Part of the Discourse I had the Honour to have with the Queen. Before I reduced it to any order I have sent it to have My Lord's Opinion what Parts I shall fix upon as fit to see the Light, by His putting a Cross before any Article'.[1] Whether on Lord Cowper's advice or for some other reason, none of the diary was ever published. Hamilton clearly did intend publication, for in a petition to George I for further royal employment he remarks that his success as a royal physician 'paroistra quant ie serer imprimer l'histoire de la maladie . . .'.[2] The diary survives in a copy made by Mary Cowper, which it seems was taken while the original version was in the possession of Lord Cowper. The original is lost, although the contents list to it has survived in the Blenheim Palace archive (see Appendix C). Suffice it to say here that the list indicates a far larger mass of material than is now available.

Hamilton's diary survives amongst the Panshanger Manuscripts at

[1] Panshanger MSS. D/EP F. 200. Three months earlier, Hamilton had shown his notes to White Kennett. This draft outlined the causes of the Queen's death and vindicated her from charges of Jacobitism. Kennett was not impressed by the latter of these two aims (Lansdowne MS. 1024, f. 470).

[2] Panshanger MSS. D/EP F. 200. Though undated, the petition was clearly written some time between the Queen's death and 15 Dec. (see p. xxiv n. 44).

Hertfordshire Record Office. There are two versions. Mary's copy, which is the basic text for this edition, consists of seventy quarto-size sheets, written in her hand on one side. At the end of the diary are copies of eight letters sent to Hamilton by the Duchess of Marlborough (see p. xliv). The second version is a generally faithful copy by Lady Sarah Cowper of her mother's draft.

If one takes Hamilton's word for it, the status of the diary as a primary source is beyond question. He insists on distinguishing 'in this my account between what I know to be true, and what I only conjecture from that knowledge'.[3] It appears from the draft of the diary (that is to say the version sent to Cowper) that Hamilton's typical approach was to record incidents and comments as soon after the event as possible and work them up subsequently either shortly afterwards or when organizing the whole narrative. He notes down whatever the Queen or others say and then glosses it with his own or others' comments. Thus typically the encounter with Godolphin (9 December 1709) gives an account of the meeting, includes direct speech from Hamilton, and notes Godolphin's acid comment. The glosses generally occur as Hamilton is writing up his notes but occasionally one sees him glossing a view at the time of composing, as when he refers on 11 May 1710 to the Queen's 'present willingness' to accept the Duchess of Marlborough's submissions. In other sections as, for example, in the opening section and the conclusion, the time of composition is clearly after the Queen's death. Or a reference to the 'Present' Lord Chancellor (23 September 1710) places the date of that area in a time after Cowper's appointment as George's Chancellor. Above all, the authentic voice of the Queen is heard frequently. Her contemptuous opinion of the Marquis of Carmarthen's statement that he was to bring over the Pretender as something spoken when he was drunk and in the night to his mistress (23 September 1710); her judgement of Sarah's daughters as being the one 'cunning and dangerous', the other 'Silly and Imprudent, and lost her Reputation', and the third, most damagingly, 'just like her Mother' (27 December 1710); and her description of the importance of Princess Sophia's death as 'Chipping-Porridge' (5 June 1714) all have a striking immediacy. Though composed by a writer sympathetic to the Whigs, the tone of the diary as we have it is never brazenly partisan and its status as an intimate document is enhanced by such balance. The aim of this edition is to present an accurate text together with some account of the diarist and the information necessary to understanding the nature of the work.

[3] Diary, p. 11.

INTRODUCTION

The Introduction is organized to give, firstly, a brief biographical account of the diarist; secondly, some information about his medical practice and his theories of medicine which appealed to the Queen; and thirdly, an analysis of his politics, his position as the Queen's confidant, and the ensuing task of go-between in the quarrel between the Queen and the Duchess of Marlborough.

1. *A Biographical Sketch of David Hamilton*

David Hamilton was born in 1663,[4] the tenth and youngest son of James Hamilton of Boggs who, on 23 August 1647, had a grant of the old Barony of Dalzell in Lanarkshire from the Earl of Carnwath and who accordingly became the first Laird of Boggs and Dalzell. His mother was Isobell, James Hamilton's third wife.[5] At the age of twenty, David Hamilton went as a medical student to the University of Leyden. He matriculated at Leyden on 30 October 1683 and judging by the annual *recensiones* he left Leyden at some stage between 15 February 1685 and 22 February 1686. It was not uncommon for medical students to go to Leyden and then proceed to another university for their degree and on 23 February 1686 Hamilton presented for his M.D. thesis at Rheims *Disputatio Medica Inauguralis de Passione Hysterica*. . . .[6] Back in England, Hamilton sought admission as a Licentiate of the College of Physicians. Having been examined by the President and Censors on 16 December 1687 and on three further occasions in January and March 1688, he was at length admitted on 9 April.[7]

On 18 July 1689 Hamilton married his first wife. She was Mary, daughter of Major Philip Starkie.[8] There were no children from the marriage and Mary died on 21 December 1691. She was buried in the church of St. Katherine Coleman, Fenchurch Street.[9] Three years later on 26 September

[4] It is difficult to establish the date of birth more precisely since the registers of the parish of Dalziel do not record births between 1661 and 1670.

[5] John Anderson, *Historical and Genealogical Memoirs of the House of Hamilton* (Edinburgh, 1825), p. 274.

[6] R. W. Innes Smith, *English-Speaking Students of Medicine at the Univ. of Leyden* (Edinburgh, 1932), p. 106, notes that this thesis is the only British Rheims thesis *pro gradu* that he was able to find.

[7] Royal College of Physicians, 'Annals'. The Annals further note that on 3 Aug. 1688, Hamilton was ordered by a Comitia Censoria to appear before it 'this Day sevennight for his ill behaviour towards Dr. Barwick'. I am grateful to the Registrar of the College for permission to quote from a contemporary transcript of the original annals. References here are to vol. v (1682–90), ff. 55b; 58a; 61a; 62b; 71a; 79a.

[8] *Register Book of The Parish of St. Christopher le Stocks*, ed. E. Freshfield. 2 vols. (1882), ii. 12.

[9] 'Register Book of the Parish of St. Katherin Coleman, London. From 25 March 1666 to

Hamilton married Elizabeth, daughter of Sir Thomas Lane (Lord Mayor of London in 1694–5).[10] There were two sons from the marriage. Thomas was christened on 26 August 1695[11] while David was born in 1700.[12]

During the 1690s and early 1700s Hamilton established a large medical practice and by his own admission accumulated considerable wealth (see p. xxviii). He also published two theological prose works, the zealous piety of which no doubt argued well for him when he was brought to the notice of Queen Anne. He was, and remained, a Dissenter[13] and published in 1697[14] and 1701[15] his personal testimonies to the effectiveness of prayer in transforming him into an ardent Christian. However, there were more practical achievements to recommend him to the Queen, notably his success in treating the Duchess of Bedford.[16] In his petition to George I[17] Hamilton observes that 'Le heureux succes que i'ay comme Medecine a l'egard de la plus part et entre austres a l'egard de la Duchesse de Bedfort ont porter la Reyne a me faire l'honneur de me choisir pour son Medecin et non pas pour son accoucher puisqu'Elle n'avoit point de tout de besoin d'une telle personne'.

His abilities were recognized in 1703. Narcissus Luttrell noted in his diary on 17 April 1703, 'The Queen has knighted Dr. Hamilton, an eminent man midwife of this citty'.[18] At the same time, he had been appointed one of the Queen's physicians-in-ordinary, and a natural reaction from the College of Physicians was that on 25 June he was 'ballotted and Elected Fellow, and admitted having subscribed the Bond upon double stampt paper for the observing the Statutes of the Colledge, and had his Diploma of

13 Sept. 1741', entry for 1691. The manuscript records are deposited at the Parish Church of St. Olave, Hart Street, with which St. Katherine Coleman amalgamated. I am grateful to the Rector for permission to use the Register Book.

[10] Guildhall Library, London, MS. 5686, entry for 1694.

[11] *The Parish Registers of St. Mary Aldermary, London, 1558–1754*. Harleian Soc. Publ., vol. 5, ed. J. L. Chester (1880), p. 111.

[12] Both sons matriculated at Oriel College, Oxford, Thomas on 20 Oct. 1713 (*Foster*, 1st ser., ii. 639), and David on 13 Apr. 1717 (*Foster*, 2nd ser., ii. 593).

[13] See pp. xxxi–ii.

[14] *The Private Christian's Witness for Christianity: In Opposition to the Notional and Erroneous Apprehensions of the Arminian, Socinian, and Deist of the Age*. A non-religious digression in this book, of interest to us, is Hamilton's reference to his 'natural disposition' which 'inclining me more to Observation, than to much Talk in Conversation, led me not only to observe the Discourse and Actions of others, but even to remark the Events attending my Life, with Reflections thereupon, without any regard to it as Duty . . . but purely as the effect of natural Curiosity . . .' (pp. 2–3).

[15] *The Inward Testimony of the Spirit of Christ To His Outward Revelation, In Opposition to the Deist, Socinian and Prophane, Who deny both . . .*

[16] The case of the Duchess is discussed in Hamilton's book on the miliary fever (see p. xxvii n. 62). The reference is to the 1737 translation, p. 43. The Duchess's husband, the second Duke, a Whig, was Lord High Constable at Anne's coronation.

[17] See p. xvii n. 2.

[18] Luttrell, v. 288.

admittance upon parchment with the double 40s, Stamp'.[19] The appointment and the knighthood roused sufficient interest to produce an indifferently written squib dated April 1703.[20] The author of the poem clearly indicates that he thinks Hamilton was called in to discover whether the Queen was pregnant or not. If the evidence of the poem is admissible, Hamilton was by 1703 both wealthy and famous. He was then rich enough to buy an estate in Lennox from the Duke of Richmond but sold it again to the Marquis of Montrose in 1704[21] after his appointment to the Queen. Though he reasoned that he would be unable to enjoy his acquisition because of his elevation, he, ironically, did not attend the Queen for some years.

His medical practice, however, flourished and in April 1708 he was elected a Fellow of the Royal Society.[22] It was at the end of 1708 that he was first called to attend upon the Queen. From then onwards, he became almost exclusively occupied with her affairs.[23] If his professional life was very successful, his private affairs were in disarray, in terms of both his health and his marriage. There are occasional references in his diary to various illnesses he suffered and consequently was unable to wait on the Queen,[24] but perhaps the most personal section of the diary occurs during December 1712. Hamilton's second marriage was not a happy one, and at this time, he was moved to speak to the Queen about his difficulties. On 10 December she, with some force one suspects, advised privacy in the matter.[25] The business was mentioned again on the 19 December and on

[19] 'Annals', vii. 204. Hamilton's name first appears on the lists of the Queen's Household as third physician. The date of the entry is 24 June 1703. No salary is recorded (PRO L.C. 3/5, f. 10).

[20] The poem exists in five versions, a remarkable indication of how well known Hamilton had become. They are Add. MS. 40060, ff. 33b–35; Add. MS. 28101, ff. 47a–48a; Stowe MS. 305, ff. 276b–277a, Bod. MS. Eng. poet., e. 50, pp. 15–18; and Nat. Lib. of Scotland, MS. 23. 2. 24., f. 95, which gives the title 'The midnight knight A Poem on the Queens knighting Doctor David Hamilton the Scots Woman Doctor'. James Boswell, whose great-grand-uncle Hamilton was, suggests that the poem was a consequence of professional jealousy (*Private Papers of James Boswell from Malahide Castle*, ed. G. Scott and F. A. Pottle, vol. 14 (1932), p. 15).

[21] For the complications of the sale, see W. Fraser, *The Earls of Cromartie Their Kindred, Country and Correspondence*, 2 vols. (Edinburgh, 1876), i. 224–8 and 255–8.

[22] *The Record of the Royal Society of London*, 4th edn. (1940), p. 391. He became a benefactor of the Society. A gift of £50 is recorded by his name on 26 June 1711 (ibid., p. 141).

[23] Hamilton's attendance at the College of Physicians was virtually non-existent for the years when he attended the Queen. From 1695 until his death in 1721, he attended only seven meetings. The last recorded instance of his being at the College was on 7 Oct. 1714, the occasion of the address to George I (Royal College of Physicians, 'Annals', viii (1711–22), 99).

[24] See, for example, the diary for 5 May to 28 Sept. 1711; 30 Jan. to 14 Feb. 1712; 20 Feb. to 5 Apr. 1712; 19 June to 6 July 1713; 9 June 1714, the last as a consequence of the news of his mother's death. His nephew, James Boswell, attended the funeral on Hamilton's behalf (*Boswell Papers*, letter for 17 June 1714). Hamilton's letters to James and Elizabeth Boswell (ibid.) con-constantly record his poor constitution.

[25] Diary, p. 45.

14 March 1713.[26] By this time others were beginning to hear the rumour circulating. Dame Sarah Cowper noted in her diary:

It struck me with Horrour to hear the story of Sr. Da— Ha— and His Lady. If what he charges Her with be True it must be own'd she is very vicious. But if what she and His Relations Accuse Him of be not false He is A most Execrable wretch. The particulars are not fit to be set down for it is a shame even to speak of those things wc. are done of them in Secret, they must be left to the Judgment of Him before whom All Things are Open and Manifest.[27]

Helena Le Grand wrote to Sir John Perceval on 24 March 1713 more explicitly:

[Sir David Hamilton] is under great uneasiness at present himself, his wife and he being parted after almost twenty year's matrimony, but she has he says given him just grounds of suspicion ever since he had been married 3 months, and daily such new proof of her infidelity that it was not safe longer for them to be together.[28]

The final reference to the sad affair is again by Dame Sarah who on 13 July 1713 cryptically observed that 'Sr. David Hamilton . . . takes Bodily pains to prove himself A Cuckold. If Either are so Bad as They tell of each other the Earth Can Bear no werse'.[29] In view of this it is not surprising that Hamilton chose to be buried with his first wife.

Like many other successful professional men of his day, Hamilton found himself with surplus capital to invest.[30] There is good evidence that he was involved in the business of the South Sea Company in the second decade of the century, and possessed some influence in its affairs, for in May 1713, he was appealed to by one Christopher Todd to support Sir Ambrose Crowley in his bid to become deputy governor.[31] Todd wonders why Hamilton, despite assurances, was making 'a strong interest' against Crowley. Whatever Hamilton's position, there is no extant evidence to support the suggestion made by a rival that Hamilton lost £80,000 in the collapse of the Company, though it is certainly true that the figure cannot be refuted, since Hamilton apparently died intestate.[32]

[26] Diary, pp. 45, 52.

[27] Dame Sarah's diaries, vi. 215–16; Panshanger MSS., D/EP F. 33 (7 Feb. 1713).

[28] Add. MS. 47027, ff. 19–20.

[29] Op. cit., p. 263.

[30] He purchased bank stock to the value of £4,600 in August and Sept., 1710; stock worth £4,500 in April and Oct., 1717, and another amount worth £5,000 in May 1719. I am grateful to the Secretary of the Bank of England for supplying me with this information.

[31] Todd to Hamilton, Wiltshire RO 79^b/4. The nature of the connection is unknown. Crowley was not elected.

[32] *DNB* (G. T. Bettany). Subsequent references to Hamilton repeat the statement (e.g. Green, *Sarah*, p. 164 n.), which derives from *Dr. Houstoun's Memoirs of his own Life-Time* (1747). Hous-

Perhaps the most remarkable single entry in the diary relating to Hamilton's personal movements occurs on 27 July 1714. The Queen proposed to send him as private envoy to Hanover 'to Settle a Sincere Friendship with the Elector' if some way might be found for him to get to Hanover without arousing suspicion.[33] Hamilton proposed to remove his son, Thomas (who had kissed the Queen's hand on 8 July 1713)[34] from Oriel College, Oxford, to either Leyden or Utrecht 'having now No familly' and thus having a valid reason to make the journey.[35] The plan was never carried out, for the Queen died on 1 August. There is perhaps no more revealing testimony about the acute crisis surrounding the Succession, than that the Queen was prepared to make use of and trust one of her physicians in so delicate a task.

As one of the royal physicians Hamilton was in attendance as the Queen was dying. He, with others, was consulted by Arbuthnot during the night of 29–30 July, and he agreed with the other doctors that, in response to the question of the Privy Council, the Queen was in a condition to be spoken to on the 30th. After her death Hamilton was a signatory to an account of the Queen's illness and the cause of death.[36]

Hamilton walked in the funeral procession of the Queen[37] and then set about the business of maintaining royal employment. In his petition to George I,[38] Hamilton contemplates with dismay 'les fausses idées que quelques uns sons doute par un principe d'interest ont tacher a luy donner de moy en luy disant, que ie n'estois qu'un accoucheur et non pas un Medecin'.[39] He evidently knew that Dr. Shadwell, who was fourth physician-in-ordinary at the time of Anne's death, enjoyed royal favour[40] for he makes it clear in the petition that he cannot be expected to serve under a physician

toun, an *accoucheur* himself, was refused help by Hamilton and his opinions were not impartial. The accuracy of this figure of £80,000 cannot be established. There are no surviving ledgers for South Sea stock or any transfer books for such stock or annuities for this period (see P. G. M. Dickson, *The Financial Revolution in England* (1967), p. 536). Boswell later defended his eminent relative from Houstoun. However, he does not refute Houstoun's figures (*Private Papers*, vol. 12, p. 67). For the legal details consequent upon Hamilton's death, see p. xxiv n. 47.

[33] Diary, p. 66.

[34] Diary, p. 57.

[35] Diary, p. 66. Thomas Hamilton did eventually go to Leyden after leaving Oxford in 1716. He was dead by March 1722 (see below, p. 112). The circumstances are a mystery.

[36] The latest account of the circumstances surrounding the Queen's death is by H. L. Snyder, 'The Last Days of Queen Anne: The Account of Sir John Evelyn Examined', *Huntington Lib. Quart.* 34 (May 1971), 261–76. See also BM Loan 29/204, f. 369; HMC *Portland MSS.* v. 483.

[37] *Cal. S.P. Dom.* 35/1, f. 75b.

[38] See p. xvii n. 2.

[39] In addition to this, there seems to have been pressure not to appoint him because he was a Dissenter. He wrote to Mary Cowper indicating that his friends were making efforts to 'Remov ill impressions as to my principles' (Panshanger MSS., D/EP F. 200; 10 Dec. 1714).

[40] Shadwell was appointed one of George's physicians in early December (*Post Boy*, 4–7 Dec. 1714). Subsequently he was 'sworn sole Physician to his Majesty' (*St. James's Post*, 9–11 Mar. 1715).

who, when Anne was alive, occupied an inferior position. Hamilton declares that 'Tout ce que mon honneur me pourroit permettre je seroit d'estre second Medecin de Vostres Majester [i.e. under George's own German doctor] ou seul aupres de la Princesse'.[41] In the latter demand Hamilton was to prove fortunate. Mary, Countess Cowper had been appointed one of the Ladies of the Bedchamber to the Princess on 28 October 1714[42] and she records in her diary for 1 November 1714 that 'Mr. B[ernstorff] made me a Visit . . . I spoke to him to desire him to take care of Sr. D.H's being made first Phisitian wch he promis'd to do . . .'.[43] She further notes on the 15 December that 'I have prevail'd for Sr. D.H. to be sole Phisitian to the P—ss'.[44] He so remained until his death in 1721, but it proved more of a sinecure than his previous post.

Hamilton died on 28 August 1721. The *Post Boy* for 26–9 August noted that he 'being ill, hath taken Lodgings near the Pond at Kensington Gravel-Pits; where Sir Hans Sloane visits him twice a day'. The same paper for 29–31 August told its readers that Hamilton 'Physician to the Prince, and eminent for Midwifry, mentioned in our last, is dead'. He was buried on Wednesday 6 September in the South Chancel of St. Katherine Coleman, Fenchurch St.[45] The *Daily Post* for 8 September reported that 'On Wednesday Night last about 12 a Clock the Corpse of the late Sir David Hamilton was interr'd very privately at St. Katherine Coleman in Fenchurch Street, where his first Wife was buryd; six Doctors held up the Pall'. A certain C. Williamson wrote a Latin elegy for Hamilton,[46] lamenting the fact that the female sex were left without the aid of Hamilton's ministering genius. Hamilton's testament was registered in Edinburgh in 1731 (3 April).[47] David, his younger son, was executor and Archibald Hamilton who had reason to be grateful for Sir David's help (See Appendix B) was the lawyer involved. The last few years of Hamilton's life remain as obscure as his youth.[48]

[41] See p. xvii n. 2.

[42] Reported in the *Daily Courant* of that date.

[43] Mary Cowper, Diary, f. 3. The Cowpers were friendly with Bernstorff and Mary acted as translator to her husband. See J. M. Beattie, *The English Court in the Reign of George I* (Cambridge, 1967), p. 145 n. 6.

[44] Ibid., f. 10. He kissed hands on the appointment in January 1715 (*Boswell Papers*, letter for 28 Jan. 1715 to James Boswell).

[45] 'Register Book of the Parish . . .', entry for 1721.

[46] BM MS. Sloane 3516, f. 188.

[47] Scottish RO., General Register House, Edinburgh. Hamilton seems not to have left a will. Letters of administration were granted to his son in Sept. 1722 (Literary Dept., Somerset House), and the testament of 1731 was a testament dative, implying that there was no will nominating an executor. A testament in Scots law signified only the confirmation of executors by the Commissary Court, in cases of intestacy.

[48] Documentation is thin for this period. There are two series of letters written while he was in

2. *Hamilton's Medical Theories and his Practice*

Hamilton was the tenth and youngest son of a relatively obscure branch of the House of Hamilton and the steps by which he became a celebrated physician throw an interesting light on the forging of a career in the late seventeenth century. His M.D. thesis on the 'hysterick passion' established his chief medical preoccupation and laid the foundation of his development as an *accoucheur*.

(i) *Theories*

As far as modern medical science is concerned, Hamilton is of no importance, except that his doctoral thesis and his diary show that he was one of a considerable number of contemporary doctors, concerned with aspects of what now would be termed psychological medicine. To argue that he was, as one writer puts it, 'centuries before his time' in psychiatry is to ignore the advances and suggestions made by Sydenham and others some years prior to Hamilton's attendance on the Queen.[49] Hamilton had indicated his interest in contemporary medical thought in his M.D. thesis for Rheims.[50] In the Preface he sympathizes with the condition of women because they are subject to greater afflictions, medically speaking, than men. The most severe of their afflictions is hysteria, affecting all ranks and ages of women and so little understood that he has chosen this ailment above all others for his chief interest and specialization in medicine. Hamilton goes on to analyse the disease, account for it, and offer his methods of cure. It seems significant that Hamilton matriculated at Leyden in 1683, the year Sydenham published his treatise on the gout, during the course of which he deals with the effects of the 'hysterick passion'.

Hamilton is concerned in his diary with two medical issues, that of the Queen's gout and the precipitation of appropriate conditions for the gout to cease to be localized and to affect other parts of the body. He argues that the 'translation' of the gout was facilitated by 'frequent returns of disquiet' which 'affected her by a gradual sinking of her Spirits and weak'ning

Bath in 1715 attempting to recover from various illnesses. One set is to Sir Hans Sloane (BM MS. Sloane 4044, ff. 102–3; 22 Oct.; 4059, ff. 100–11; April to Sept.: ff. 108–11 for Feb. and June 1716 were written when he returned to London). The other set is to Mary Cowper and provides an interesting commentary on the West country, especially Bath and Bristol, at the time of the Rebellion (Panshanger MSS. D/EP F. 200). Apart from this, there remain some brief letters to Scotland (see Appendix B) and three further letters to Mary Cowper of 1718 and early 1719 (Panshanger MSS. D/EP F. 200).

[49] D. Green, *Queen Anne* (1970), p. 205.

[50] See p. xix. I am grateful to Miss Helen Reed of the Dept. of Classics, University of Newcastle, for providing me with a translation of the Latin text.

of her nerves'. These 'translations' occur particularly during the condition known as 'Vapours'.[51] Such a condition (subsequently called by Cheyne 'the English malady') was applied to all kinds of depressive illnesses for centuries. The ancient medical world related it to the movement of the womb, and it was not until the second half of the seventeenth century that this uterine physiology began to be modified. Thomas Willis (1667) placed the pathology of the complaint in 'the Brain and Nervous Stock' and liberated the uterus (and with it the 'humours') from being the cause of depression or hysteria.[52] Willis postulated a disturbance of the brain and nerves in terms of disordered 'Animal Spirits' which were thought to be distilled from the blood in the brain, their circulation accounting for nervous action. In so far as these spirits act as intermediaries between mind and body, they provide the exact basis for Hamilton's notions of the nerves being weakened by disquiet, thus enabling the physical disease, the gout, to wreak a physical effect. Hamilton, as did others, recognized and attempted to treat the mental manifestations of the disease. He took seriously a complaint which rapidly became fashionable. Dr. Radcliffe characteristically had refused on one occasion to take Princess Anne's complaint seriously. On being sent for in 1694, he remarked that 'Her Highness's distemper was nothing but the vapours, and she was in as good a state of health as any woman breathing . . .'.[53] Radcliffe was dismissed the following day and on becoming Queen, Anne resisted all appeals for his reinstatement.[54] It is a fairly safe assumption that Hamilton's appointment was at least partly to do with his growing eminence as a specialist in female afflictions.

Before Hamilton, Thomas Sydenham had dealt more specifically with the problem of gout, even though in this connection he reverts basically to a humoral doctrine.[55] He notes the inevitability of the delocalization of the gout for 'this translation of the humours occasioning the *gout* and forming a *gouty* fit happens sooner or later, according as these humours are occasionally put in motion'.[56] Sydenham links such an occurrence with weakened 'spirits': To these observations must be added, that the same paucity of spirits which hurts

[51] Diary, p. 3.

[52] Some of this section derives from R. Hunter and I. Macalpine, *Three Hundred Years of Psychiatry 1535–1860* (O.U.P., 1963). Here the reference is to pp. 187–8.

[53] C. R. Hone, *The Life of Dr. John Radcliffe 1652–1714* (1950), p. 51.

[54] Ibid. See Diary, p. 31.

[55] It should be made clear that the diagnosis of what was generally known as 'gout' was in the context of humoral pathology. It was classed as a catarrh and was thought to be caused by a liquid secretion which was distilled drop by drop on the diseased part (see H. A. Skinner, *The Origins of Medical Terms* (Baltimore, 1961), pp. 195–6).

[56] *Tractatus de Podagra et de Hydrope* (1683). Swan's translation of 1742 in *Selected Works of . . . Sydenham*, ed. J. D. Comrie (1922), p. 67.

the concoctions in *gouty* subjects renders their spirits weak and languid, so that they are soon disturbed by any course which considerably hurries either the body or mind, and consequently are very volatile and dissipable, as they frequently are in *hysteric* and *hypochondriac* patients.[57]

Sydenham's advised course of action foreshadows Hamilton's constant advice to the Queen when he argues that 'The patient must likewise use his utmost endeavour to keep his mind easy, for all disquieting passions, if they once become immoderate, greatly dissolve the texture of the spirits, which are the instruments of digestion, and so of course increase the gout'.[58] Hamilton's opinions of the Queen's illnesses and his course of action were not only consistent with the views of Sydenham but his view of the cause of death was shared by those others of the Queen's physicians whose opinions are extant. Arbuthnot felt that the Queen's struggle with conflicting rights and duties brought her prematurely to the grave[59] and Shadwell's opinion was reported by Boyer that quarrelling among the Queen's servants produced the remark that '*She should not outlive it*'. The dispute occasioned 'such a violent Agitation of the Queen's Spirits, as could not but hinder the *usual Discharge of the Impostumation in her Leg; so that the gouty Humour translating it self upon the Brain, was the immediate Occasion of her Death*'.[60]

(ii) *Practice*

In his later career, Hamilton was at pains to deny that his ability rested principally on his skills as an *accoucheur*, and his petition to George I traced his career,[61] insisting that after leaving Rheims, he had no thought of becoming a midwife: 'Mais ensuitte estant retourner de Rheims a Paris et ayant fait reflexion, que la partie de la medecine la moins cultivée estoit cells qui traitte des maladies des femmes dont il est impossible d'avoir une juste connoissance sans avoir celle d'accoucheur . . .' Despite his disavowal, he was nevertheless more celebrated as a midwife than for any other branch of medicine with the sole exception of his treatment of the miliary fever.[62] In the same petition, Hamilton notes his good fortune with only a minimum

[57] Ibid., p. 69.

[58] Ibid., pp. 85–6.

[59] Strickland, viii. 538.

[60] Boyer, *Annals* (1722 edn.), p. 714.

[61] See p. xvii n. 2. Some idea of his reputation as both midwife and general specialist in feminine maladies may be gained by reference to the papers of James Douglas in the Hunterian Library, University of Glasgow. I am grateful to Mr. C. H. Brock of the Dept. of History of Science for drawing my attention to these items, which refer mainly to the years 1701–7.

[62] His account of this disease was published in 1710 (*Tractatus Duplex Prior de Praxeos Regulis Alter de Febri Miliari*, 1710). The book which was dedicated to the Queen became the definitive work for some time. George Cheyne testified to Hamilton's expertise in treating the fever (*The Cure of the Miliary Fever* . . . (1751), pp. vii–viii, note a), while other doctors wrote to ask him for his advice (BM MS. Sloane 4075, ff. 349–50).

of exaggeration: 'La providence de Dieu a aussi concouru avec moy la dedans, m'ayant donné depuis l'age de vingt et deux ans une practique plus estendre qu'aucun Medecine ait peut estre jamais eu non obstant la malice et l'envie de plusieurs.'

In the five and a half years between Hamilton's appointment as a royal physician and his being called to attend the Queen, Anne clearly had no use for his talent as a midwife, and it could be that she only ultimately recalled him when he might prove useful in the handling of her estrangement from the Duchess of Marlborough (see p. xxxii ff.). Meanwhile, Hamilton's private practice had remained healthy. Lady Pye noted in a letter to Abigail Harley on 15 January 1707 that 'Sr. David Hambleton, had better success with my neighbor Mrs. Wilmote who went to lye in with her Mother La Marrow, lay near 3 day's but both Mother & child like to do well'.[63] He was highly thought of by others, including the Herveys. There are frequent references to his skills by Lady Hervey regarding her own delicate health and that of her son, James. Hamilton delivered Lady Hervey's tenth son in February 1712 and remained her personal physician until his death in 1721.[64] However, clear disaster was the consequence of his attendance on the wife of the sixth Earl of Westmorland who in 1708 had married the daughter of Thomas Stringer. Hamilton was sent for from London and attempted to induce the child by having the Earl's wife driven in a coach over some very rough roads.

> which he did for about an hour to her great Missery & then Comeing home found it not to Answer his Purpose being more greedy for his money than Mindfull of his duty he hurryed away as aforesd . . . I understood by words he had droped, that he was sensible he had done her an injury not only to the Present Child but also to future expectations, & so it hath Proved for from that time the Child never stirred . . . this I Note that the Villany may be remember'd to avoid the like.[65]

Hamilton remained third physician to Queen Anne until 2 February 1712, at which point the death of Dr. Lister made room for his promotion to second physician.[66] He appears to have felt somewhat cheated by Anne's

[63] BM Loan 29/194, f. 10; HMC *Portland MSS*. iv. 382.

[64] *The Diary of John Hervey* . . . (Wells, 1894), p. 56 (12 Feb. 1712); *Letter-Books of John Hervey, First Earl of Bristol* . . . *1651–1750*, 3 vols. (Wells, 1894), i. 362, 365, 368–71; ii. 5–6, 85, 129–30, 136, 141, 142, etc.

[65] Add. MS. 34223, ff. 32b–34 (Westmorland's Memoirs); HMC *Westmorland MSS*. iv. 52.

[66] He was officially sworn in on 17 February. The document survives and is an interesting example of Household ceremonial (Bod. MSS. Rawl. A. 289, f. 220). Details of Hamilton's salary may be found in: John Chamberlayne, *Magnae Britanniae Notitia* . . ., 23rd edn., p. 543; *Cal. Treas. Bks.* xxvii (pt. 2), 517; xxviii (pt. 2), 257, 372; PRO L.C. 3/6, f. 10. See also Diary, p. 56 (6 July 1713), and his memorial for arrears of pay in 1715 (*Cal. Treas. Papers*, cxcvi. 11, 171).

death, for one of the points he makes in his petition to George I[67] is that he aspired to a higher position and that 'la justice de Vostre Majester . . . n'exigera pas de moy qu'aupres avoir ester sur le point d'estre premier Medecin de . . . la Reyne ie sois comme simple accoucheur de le Princesse Royale'.

Having been appointed physician to the Princess, he attended her in her labour of 1716. She had not been well since the middle of the year, for Lady Cowper told Mrs. Clayton that 'The Princess has been mightily out of order. She was in great danger of miscarrying . . . She has taken some things Sir David Hamilton gave her, and I hope she is out of danger for this time, though I wish she would take a little more care of herself'.[68] Despite his protests in his petition to George I Hamilton once more figured centrally as an *accoucheur* or rather would have done so had he been allowed to attend the Princess. Mary Cowper wrote on 4 November that

> ye Princess fell into Labour upon wch ye Council was call'd. there was a German Midwife (whose countenance prognosticated Ill, she being ye very Picture of ye French Resident) & Sr David Ham: waited as Phisitian . . . ye English Ladys all press'd to have ye Ps. laid by Sr D. but she woud not hear of it . . .[69] we all ask'd Sr D. who sd he apprehended ye Child come on one side ye head wch might be easily help'd by a Skilful hand, but wd infallibly kill ye Child if not prevented.[70]

Throughout the week Mary and others made attempts to gain entry for Hamilton, for the midwife was 'a poor ignorant Creature . . .'.[71] Mary reported 'ye Council to send down for ye Countess of Piquebourg to desire her to let ye Prince know yt they were there to beseech him to perswade the Princess to be Ld by Sr D. wch he was angry at'.[72]

By the middle of the week the view was that the Princess was carrying a dead child and Mary seems representative of general opinion when she says that the child 'had infallibly been alive if she had been laid by Sr D.H'.[73] Apart from quarrelling with other doctors and watching the German midwife

[67] See p. xvii n. 2.

[68] *Memoirs of Viscountess Sundon*, ed. Mrs. Thomson, 2 vols. (1847), i. 334 (18 Aug. 1716).

[69] Caroline's biographer gives the reason for this as 'misplaced modesty' (R. L. Arkell, *Caroline of Ansbach* (O.U.P., 1939), p. 95).

[70] Mary Cowper, Diary f. 68 (4 Nov.).

[71] Ibid.

[72] Ibid. The Prince told the Dukes of Bolton and St. Albans that he would fling any meddlers out of the window (Arkell, op. cit., p. 96).

[73] Mary Cowper, Diary, f. 69. Dudley Ryder's opinion was the same: 'It was said by Dr. Hollier and most people that she might have been delivered the Tuesday before of a live child if she would have made use of Sir David Hamilton and suffered herself to be laid then, but she refused both' (*The Diary of Dudley Ryder 1715–1716*. Transcr. and ed. by W. Matthews (1939), p. 363; 13 Nov. 1716). Sir Gustavus Hume vigorously agreed (HMC Polwarth MSS. I, 141; to Lord Polwarth, 30 Nov. 1716).

becoming flustered, Hamilton did little else while in attendance except eat.[74]

A year later, the Princess again was in labour. Hamilton was again in attendance but was sufficiently underemployed to be requisitioned from the royal bedside to attend the Duchess of Argyle who was three days in labour.[75] The Princess, however, was not well. The circumstances following the birth of the Duke of Gloucester (who died in infancy) are described in Stratford's letters to Edward Harley.[76] The Princess clearly regarded Hamilton with some affection as witness Hamilton's remarks in a letter to Mary Cowper that he 'was surprisd with the goodness of the princess, offering of herself to write to princ Frederick with Tom [his son], and to acquaint him he was the Son of him who had saved here Life'.[77]

Although Hamilton constantly asserted throughout his career that he was more than a midwife, all the newspapers when reporting the fact of his death characterized him as pre-eminently skilled in midwifery.[78] He would perhaps have been pleased to find that Lady Bristol, who was inconsolable over his death, saw his medical talents ranging wider than the newspaper obituaries. Her words provide a fitting epitaph for Hamilton the physician. Her husband, John Hervey, wrote on 30 August 1721: 'I heartily condole with you upon the death of Sir D. Hamilton; but thanks be to God, all skill in womens waies are not departed with him; besides I trust in his goodness that you may never have any future need of any . . .'. She replied on 2 September that his death was 'a cutting stroak to one in my condition to loose the cheif (nay only) assistance I depended on to recover my ill state of health; I dare not tell you all the aprehensions it has given to my weak and depressd spirits . . .'.[79]

[74] Details of this are in a manuscript, 'Bills of Fare for their Royal Highnesses the Prince and Princess of Wales . . .' (1715–16), now in the possession of Kenneth Monkman, Esq., who has kindly supplied me with the relevant information. Hamilton was served an 'extraordinary' meal from 6–11 Nov.: 'on the 6th he had only a roast chicken; on the 7th a loin of mutton; on the 8th Pottage [and] Pullet rost . . . 1; on the 9th Chicken wh. Oysters . . . 2; on the 10th Beef bo[iled] . . . 1. Partridge bd sauce . . . 1; and on the 11th Chicken with Oysters . . . 2. Breast Veale, swttdb . . . 1.'

[75] BM Loan 29/204, f. 78, Dr. Stratford to Edward Harley, 14 Nov. 1717; HMC *Portland MSS.* v. 536–7.

[76] Ibid. 29/204, f. 95; HMC *Portland MSS.* v. 546; 29/204, f. 96; HMC *Portland MSS.* v. 548.

[77] Panshanger MSS. D/EP F. 200. The letter is undated but almost certainly refers either to this confinement or possibly to that in 1716. The same letter indicates the Princess's resolution not to choose nurses without the benefit of Hamilton's advice.

[78] See, for example, the *Weekly Journal or Saturday's Post* for 2 Sept. 1721; *Weekly Journal or British Gazetteer* for the same date; *Daily Post* for 29 Aug. *Applebee's Original Weekly Journal* for 2 Sept. remarked knowingly that he was 'famous in the Practice of Midwifry, and, as some say, in another Practice also. He is like to be much miss'd among the Female Sex'.

[79] Hervey, *Letter-Books*, ii. 175, 178. Hervey noted the death of 'an honest North-Briton' (*The Diary of John Hervey* . . ., p. 71).

3. *Hamilton in Politics: Whig, Royal Confidant, and Political Broker*

Hamilton's chief preoccupation, according to the diary, was to do with the Queen's health and the cumulative effects of anxiety upon her constitution. However, it is apparent from the diary that Hamilton's inclinations in politics were Whig. His friends and contacts mentioned most often in his account are strong Whigs, whilst he clearly distrusts Harley. Yet he was no fanatic nor was he at all enamoured of what he describes as 'Party-heat'.[80] Part of the reason for this aversion was its effect upon the Queen. After the Queen was dead he remarked apropos of the 1715 uprising that his anger at the Rebellion was 'contrary to my natural calmness of temper and habitual moderation in party matters but its [the anger] from good ground and not from fancy and built upon rational certainty'.[81] His dissenting beliefs would naturally not incline him towards the Tories. In a revealing letter to Mary[82] he refers to the fourth Occasional Conformity Bill (1711) and says:

> I woud sugest one thing I never thought off that when the ocasionale bill past I would hav Layd down but that my Lord [Cowper] hindered me by saying that then they should hav not a faithful servant of her health or gett any other Service done upon which I hav payd yearly ever since a hundred pound a year for 2 to preach in my own house and continued this becaus if I shoud be seen once a meetting I should not be capable of being in any post in the family . . .

Hamilton was thus for the Whigs in valuable proximity to the Queen and at least part of his importance for them was that he would regularly present to her views other than those of the ministry.[83] He was in a prime position to convey information, comment, and opinion to the Queen from Cowper, Godolphin, and others out of office. As well as becoming the main channel of information and letters from the Duchess of Marlborough, he arranged appointments for Cowper[84] and was the means whereby Godolphin wrote his advice to the Queen on 27 December 1710 regarding the necessity for

[80] Diary, p. 10. Both of his sons were, however, more zealous. Thomas and David were involved in riots surrounding the meetings of the Whig Constitutional Club in Oxford (Panshanger MSS. D/EP F. 200; BM Loan 29/227, f. 444, Stratford to Harley, 30 May 1717).

[81] Panshanger MSS. D/EP F. 200; To Mary Cowper (15 Oct. 1715).

[82] Ibid.; undated but probably at the end of 1714, when he sought employment with the Princess of Wales.

[83] Such occasions are frequent in the diary. The entry for 12 Sept. 1710 is typical. It is worth pointing out that Hamilton became increasingly important to the Whigs as, first, the Duke of Newcastle went out (July 1711) and, second, the Duke of Somerset (Jan. 1712). After this, only the Duchess of Somerset retained a similar intimacy with Anne as Hamilton. The densest and most documented parts of the diary are the sections covering 1711 and 1712.

[84] The former Chancellor's pocket diaries record Hamilton's name on lists of appointments in 1711 and 1712 (Panshanger MSS. D/EP F. 71–8).

supporting the alliance for the recovery of Spain.[85] Harley of course recognized the danger and indeed made attempts to get Hamilton out. The following reference would suggest that the Occasional Conformity Bill gave him his opportunity, for Hamilton maintained in his petition to George that he was most successful as the Queen's physician 'et c'est a cause de cela aussi qu'Elle ne voulut jamais consentir a m'eloigner d'Elle quoi que My Lord Oxford la pressat fort la dessus il y a deux ans.'[86] Hamilton was ready to lay down in 1711, Harley was pressing him so to do, but he stayed as a consequence of Whig appeals.

Nevertheless the issue for Hamilton was not based upon party. For his concern was with the Queen and his constant point of reference is not to the efficacy or otherwise of such and such a measure (although he does on occasions express an opinion) but to the effect of any event upon his royal mistress. 'My Business is only to Vindicate her that is gone' he asserts in the diary for 15 June 1710 and this vindication is the mainspring of his concerns. His fidelity received its sternest test in the business concerning the Duchess of Marlborough. The fact of the estrangement of Queen Anne and the Duchess of Marlborough is well enough known and needs no detailed repetition. What has not been known until now are the precise steps by which the Duchess came to lay down her offices in January 1711. Hamilton's diary shows the vital degree to which he became the chief negotiator and go-between in the handling of what became, especially for the Queen during 1710, a potentially explosive issue. Between 4 April 1710 and 18 January 1711, Hamilton conversed with Anne some fifty-five times about the threats, pleadings, and complaints of the Duchess of Marlborough. His part in the affair, evidence of which occurs in the diary and elsewhere, is an index of his importance to the Queen and her trust in his abilities. His influence has received scant attention until now.[87]

It was Hamilton who was partly responsible for persuading the Queen to keep Sarah in until the Duke returned at the end of 1710 and who, in so far as anyone could, reduced Sarah's impetuosity to a minimum. He reported to the Queen as much of what Sarah wrote and said as was commensurate

[85] See Appendix D. The letter had originally been sent to the Cowpers on 18 Mar. 1715 together with the diary and other material.

[86] See p. xvii n. 2.

[87] Most of the printed sources take their information from Coxe (iii. 169–72, 175) and make the general point about Hamilton as an intermediary. Thus F. W. Wyon, *The History of Great Britain during the Reign of Queen Anne*, 2 vols. (1876), ii. 264–6; Strickland, viii. 386–9 (for whom Hamilton is the 'physician-spy'); M. R. Hopkinson, *Anne of England* (1934), p. 310; and N. Connell, *Anne The Last Stuart Monarch* (1937), pp. 230, 237. Recently the account has been repeated by Green, *Sarah*, pp. 163–4, 323, and more elaborately, in *Queen Anne* (1970).

with his medical opinion of Anne's health and he reported to Sarah as many of the Queen's feelings as were calculated to soothe the meteoric temper of the Duchess. To do so required no mean diplomatic ingenuity for he must have known that a rearguard action was the only strategy proper to a battle which in effect from Sarah's point of view was clearly lost. From April 1710 up to and beyond Sarah's going out, Hamilton was saddled with a responsibility far beyond his position but, ironically, a responsibility which came about only because of his position, which afforded a proximity to the Queen unavailable to others who might be sympathetic to Sarah's cause. The following account sets the diary in the context of Sarah's thoughts and activities during 1710 and perhaps shows how her eventual dismissal was bound up with the steady erosion of Godolphin's administration by Harley.

The diary commences at the beginning of December 1709. While Hamilton plainly states that he can say nothing of the estrangement 'but from the Time her Majesty commanded me to wait upon her Grace, to convey her pleasure to the Dutchess and her answers to the Queen',[88] the diary nevertheless begins to record matters connected with the quarrel and with the gradual emergence of measures taken against the Godolphin ministry. It was during the series of attempts Sarah made to see the Queen from 3 to 6 April, culminating in the final interview on the 6th that the Queen, on 4 April, 'then committed the affair to me; with which also my Lord Godolphin seemd extreamly pleas'd, promising to write for the Duchess, who was then at Windsor, on purpose that I might speak to her'. What emerges from the entry for 4 April (which appears to be a composite entry covering several days) is that the affair had reached crisis point and that the Queen had been unwilling to part with Godolphin as the inevitable consequence of dismissing Sarah. Accordingly she had instructed Hamilton to tell Godolphin to influence Sarah 'to make her submissions'. Sarah, however, came to the Queen before Godolphin had seen her and as a result, the Queen decided it was useless for Godolphin to see Sarah and, it being clear that the breach was final, Hamilton was given his instructions. In an undated memorandum, Hamilton recorded his impression of what subsequently developed from this point up to the dismissal of the Duchess:

1. to shew the Queen's order to me to endeavour to bring her to make her submission because of her unwillingness to part with my Lord Godolphin wch she was made to believe was of necessity if my Lady Marlborough was put out.

[88] Diary, p. 4.

2. her reseding from that, from their convincing her of the necessity of parting with my Lord Godolphin as what wou'd give her uneasiness instead of quiet
3. my conversing with my Lady Marlborough upon the subject of vindicating her self and accusing the Queen, my reporting to the Queen what she said, and reading what she wrote to me upon that subject, and reporting to the Dutchess of Marlborough the Queen's answers, in which is included, Lady Marlborough's accusing the Queen with breach of promises with asseverations, my endeavour with divines to know the strength of that accusation, and laying it before the Queen; the Dutchess of Marlborough's threatning her, with printing her letters wrote under the power of her affection then to her, the Queen's answer and my successful use of that threatning as a mean, of not turning her out disgracfully till my Lord Marlborough return'd and then to order it that she shou'd rather give up the Key.[89]

The reasons for which the affair was entrusted to Hamilton are not clear. Coxe's suggestion that Hamilton owed his appointment as a royal physician to Sarah's patronage[90] will not hold when Sarah so obviously was not sure about this latest emissary from the Queen. Hamilton's brief initially involved a holding operation in order to enable the Queen to keep Godolphin in and subsequently his brief was one of delaying or preventing the printing of the Queen's letters and investigating the strength of her promises to Sarah once Godolphin had been put out. As a Whig he could be expected to be received by Sarah with some degree of warmth but as the Queen's physician, as he often says, his primary duty was to the Queen's health. His being given the task might simply have been on the basis that there was no one else to be sent to Sarah or to whom Sarah would speak in confidence amongst those currently surrounding the Queen. He did, after all, offer a direct avenue of access to the Queen and he was not, as far as the Whigs knew, being suborned by Harley. A man trusted by the Cowpers might be supposed to be worthy of some conversation with the Duchess of Marlborough.

After her last meeting with the Queen, Sarah left town and resisted appeals to return.[91] Despite Godolphin's writing several times to secure an appointment for him, Hamilton was not to have the interview with Sarah until rumours of Sunderland's dismissal began to be circulated in early June. Meanwhile he had been faced with the Queen's difficulties, for the diary records her concern at finding that the removal of Godolphin could well follow Sarah's departure (4 April). The pressure to remove Godolphin increased, but his apparent readiness to accept without demur the appoint-

[89] Bod. MSS. Rawl. D. 924, f. 516 (in Hamilton's hand).

[90] iii. 169.

[91] The Duke, before leaving England in February 1710, had secured the Queen's permission for Sarah to stay in the country as much as possible (Coxe, iii. 52).

ment of Shrewsbury (14 April) pleased the Queen as did the proposed interview of Hamilton with Sarah, which however Sarah was proving reluctant to grant throughout April and May. It was in May that the Queen tried to effect a separation between Sarah and Godolphin via Hamilton, but the intimacy was too strong for that. Sarah stayed doggedly out of London and resisted appeals to return.[92]

In June, Sarah came quickly from the country upon the rumours of Sunderland's dismissal. Hamilton then finally managed to see her and related the interview to the Queen on 15 June. The Duchess justified herself to Hamilton and reacted with indignation to the criticism that she argued with the Queen by letter. Interestingly it was she who raised the question of finance at this point, a topic soon to be capitalized on by Swift. In the *Conduct*, Sarah refers to Hamilton as follows:

The same necessity which forced her MAJESTY to dismiss my lord GODOLPHIN from her service, rendered her irreconcilable to me, though by means of one person at court, who happened to be in good favour with her, I made all possible attempts to remove her unjust prejudices against me. I wrote to him long and plain accounts of what had past, justifying myself, and exposing the ingratitude as well as malice of my enemies: All which accounts he read to the QUEEN, but without any effect upon her . . .[93]

Sarah noted elsewhere her understanding of Hamilton's task. She endorsed her copy of a letter to him with:

a copy of a leter of lady marlboroughs written to a person the queen Employd some times to goe to her out of curiosity to hear what she said & lady marl: had reason to think this person endeavourd to doe good offices thinking it for the queens service to sett all things right, & hee told lady marl: that hee allways read any thing she writt to him to the q: that hee thought might bee of use but never told her that lady marl: knew that, & the queen incouraged him to tell her all hee heard by which means la: marl: could write to him as a friend what could not bee said to the queen, this correspondence between lady marl: & this person I think did begin tell a little before or after my Ld sunderland was removed from being secretary of state in June 1710.[94]

In one of the first letters Sarah wrote to the Queen she gave her assent to the use of Hamilton as envoy. She apologized to the Queen 'if I humbly presume to approach you in this manner, there being now no other way left for me, or any other person without being too much exposed to the

[92] Mary Cowper to Sarah, 14 May (*Priv. Corr.* i. 313); Marlborough to Sarah, 29 May (ibid. i. 327).
[93] *Conduct*, p. 263.
[94] Blenheim MSS. G-I-8 (in Sarah's hand).

observation & malice of those about you . . .'.[95] However, just as Hamilton was cautious in what he read to the Queen,[96] Sarah was equally cautious in her dealings with him, for

the queen Employd this man to come to me, & hee said to me that nothing had any Effect upon her but flattry, or fear, & for that reason he tryd to fright her about the leters I had in my power told her often that hee did protest hee woud not fall out with any body that might doe him such hurt, & upon his saying to her that hee feard my provocations might make me print her leters for I had a very high spirit, & it was by her order that hee writt a leter to me at Windsor . . . & hee was to write as a friend from him self to prevent my doing any thing that might reflect upon her, which was the occasion of severall of these leters in which I took care to make her think hee had great interest with me, & that hee loved her extreamly that hee might bee more likely to Effect any thing that was for her good as well as my own for she saw every thing I writt . . . & she thought I knew nothing of her seeing the leters which hee orderd in that manner that I might say what could not otherwise have been told to a q;[97]

What appears evident from this is that all of those concerned were sure that they knew the whole picture but that David Hamilton knew more than most. Sarah's opinion of Hamilton fluctuated. She initially believed him to be sincere and honest, though biased in favour of the Queen. Hamilton 'has so good a Character that I durst trust Him with the whole truth'.[98] When, however, the Duke of Marlborough visited the Queen on Hamilton's recommendation, a visit which terminated with Sarah's dismissal, the Duchess made the general comment that 'it was Sr David Hamilton who had opertunitys of seeing her alone every day & as hee asured me hee read several of my leters to the queen & tho hee was not an honest man I believe hee spoke the truth in this because what hee repeated of the queen was allways very like her . . .'.[99] When Sarah came to compose the drafts of what became the *Conduct*, she appears to have had difficulty in deciding how to signify Hamilton's part. In one draft he appears as 'a friend'. In another, he is 'One person at Court, who was now in good favour with ye *Queen* [who] made what attempts He could, to soften matters between them, if not to heal them'. In another, he is 'a friend that had frequent opportunitys of talking with the Queen'. In yet another, Hamilton figures as 'the Gentleman' and 'a friend'.[100] In the published version of the *Conduct* he is simply 'one person at court'. If her

95 Ibid. G-I-16 (fair copy).

96 According to the diary, Hamilton read at least nine of Sarah's letters to the Queen. Coxe notes rightly that copies of Sarah's letters to Hamilton, if published, would fill a volume (iii. 169).

97 Blenheim MSS. G-I-8 (Sarah's hand).

98 Ibid. (a fair copy, possibly to Maynwaring).

99 Ibid. (Sarah's hand).

100 Ibid. G-I-9; G-I-9; G-I-10; and G-I-16 respectively.

feelings towards Hamilton were subject to change, it remains the case that, from April 1710 to the end of the year, he provided the main opportunity of contacting the Queen other than through official channels. Sarah had no choice in the matter.

After the first interview reported to the Queen on 15 June, Hamilton saw Sarah only once during the rest of June (19th). She had left town and was reportedly furious over Sunderland's being put out. In June the long series of letters to Hamilton began, the formulation of which was to provide the basis for the *Conduct*. A typical piece is in response to Hamilton's initial inquiries as to her grievances and begins: 'I have given you an account of what you seem'd most desirous to know concerning the particulars in which I have been very much wrong'd, & now I have a mind to put down some facts concerning these poor relations of mine. . . .'[101] The threat to print the Queen's letters was revived as a weapon by Sarah at the end of June and the beginning of July. She wrote asking Hamilton 'to get her promise that when she has read two or three of her own leters to me, or perhaps more, which I will send you for her, that she will give you her word before hand that she will send them me again, for those I am resolved I will not part with whatever course she would take to have them . . .'.[102] Sarah began to gather her papers together in order to write her vindication. On 26 June she wrote to Maynwaring and referred to Hamilton under the cipher of '260':

> I found the inclosed paper after I writt to you yesterday, which is a part of the famous history that is to bee, which 260 did not see & I have a great many other wonderfull things that must bee broughte in, but I writt them generally as they happen, & they are laid up very carefully, in different places, I wish you would shew 260 this because it will not only prove a very extraordinary proceeding, but it will shew what I writt to the q; in hopes to have saved my lord marl: the trouble of seeing his son turnd out . . . if 260 cares for a coppy of this hee may take it, for tis all true . . .[103]

Her intense activity in June brought a fervent appeal from the Duke that, given the Queen's attitude, '39 begs of 240 that she will not, on any account, be prevailed upon to write any more to the Queen; and I should think the prudent behaviour for 240 should be, not to be in the way of being solicited'.[104] But Sarah was in no mood to keep quiet, especially with Hamilton providing a ready way for her to write to the Queen. While that was available

[101] Ibid. G-I-8 (fair copy).

[102] Ibid. (Sarah's hand).

[103] Ibid. (Sarah's hand). Maynwaring knew Hamilton, for he refers briefly to him in a letter to Sarah (Blenheim MSS. E-29).

[104] *Priv. Corr.* i. 354 (30 June).

she no doubt felt a chance, however remote, of changing events but taking that route actually ensured that energy was dissipated which might have found more ominous outlets.

Sarah was back in town by 8 July for Hamilton informed the Queen of the fact and relayed the printing threat. He felt at this point that the removal of Sarah was being contemplated for he urged the Queen to do it 'in a way the least provoking'. The Duchess began to raise the question of the Queen's promise of her places going to her children and this issue was to form a vital part of the proceedings for the rest of 1710. As yet it is raised only briefly on 10 July, as also the suggestion that Sarah not be put out until Marlborough himself goes out. Sarah, according to Hamilton's entry for the 10th, was both threatening the Queen and giving her an alternative by which Sarah would stay in and keep quiet. For the rest of the month the Queen said nothing of the Duchess and read without comment a letter sent by Sarah to Hamilton on 28 July, the first of Sarah's letters which he handed over to the Queen. Sarah absented herself from town for the latter part of July, and the first two and a half weeks of August. She maintained an ominous silence as Godolphin was put out and replaced by a Harleyite Treasury Board. She then spoke to Hamilton on the 18th and complained bitterly of the manner in which Godolphin was dismissed. It seems as if Sarah had decided that the time of her own dismissal was nearing, and she attempted to see the Queen who, on 23 August, carefully avoided an inevitable repetition of 6 April in ordering Hamilton to shield her by going to see what the Duchess had to say. Marlborough at this time urged caution in writing to Sarah and begged her to keep out of the way of providing an opportunity for removal.[105] But by the time he had so written, Sarah had gone to town. Hamilton visited her on 24 August and was told not to trust the Queen for she broke her promises regarding Sarah's children. This issue became a central one. Sarah perhaps recognized that she must go, and wished to; yet she still tried, arguably foolishly, to ensure that her children received her places. Or it may be more likely the case that even Sarah realized the impossibility of such an event but reckoned it as a method whereby she might stay in until the Duke returned, thus avoiding further mortifications to him. Prophetically, Marlborough said that 'as soon as the winter comes, they will put in execution what they have so unjustly designed . . .'.[106]

In September Sarah told Hamilton forcefully about the promise. On the 16th he confronted the Queen with this matter, which was to trouble him apparently on a question of principle rather more than it troubled Anne.

[105] Ibid. i. 366 (28 Aug.); i. 367 (30 Aug.). [106] Ibid. i. 378 (18 Sept.).

The Queen seemed to evade the issue by saying 'that persons may Promise, and yet upon Occurrences change . . .'. Yet Sarah insisted a written promise had been made by the Queen.[107] The strong likelihood of this letter being real and not a figment or misinterpretation on Sarah's part is confirmed by the vehemence with which she pursued the matter and the equivocation with which the Queen met the challenge. It certainly worried Hamilton who wrote to Sarah rather weakly inquiring after the strength of the promise. Sarah sent a strong reply:

you wished that I could propose any Expedient to you that might ease the Q. in that particular, I shou'd be willing if Her Ma:tie lik't it to refer that & this whole matter to any Clergyman of a good reputation, & wou'd positively do whatever he thought fit for me, With Regard to this World & the next . . . it is more for her Ma:ties honour & Service that I shou'd leave her in an naturall way with Ld. Marlb: which will Save the q: from all manner of uneasyness, Whereas I do really think if what is talkt of is put in Execution after such expressions under ye q's *own hand*, It will bring such Reflections upon her Ma:tie As I wish never to see . . .[108]

Sarah later commented on the Queen's refusal of the offer of arbitration that 'she asked [Hamilton] if hee had seen those letters, to wch he answerd, Yes, & upon that she looks thoughtfull, but the next day told Him she lookt upon all those promises to be at an End, when the person to whom they were made was undutyfull . . .'.[109]

The business hung fire for the time being. The chief Whig lords resigned or were dismissed, Parliament was dissolved on 21 September, and events were moving inexorably into the last phase as far as Sarah was concerned. The diary for October observes very little while the Whigs were suffering a great defeat in the general election. Hamilton was in intermittent contact with Sarah and read a letter of hers to the Queen on the 30th. On Hamilton's advice Sarah kept quiet for most of October and November but explosively reacted to Swift's famous *Examiner* no. 17, published on 23 November, accusing the Marlboroughs of salting away public funds. She defended herself via Hamilton, who relayed the letter to the Queen on 29 November. The Queen recognized that Sarah's mood was such that the threat of a public vindication might become a reality, for on 30 November Hamilton records her talking of attempting to regain her letters to Sarah, and musing on the

[107] Blenheim MSS. G-I-7; Coxe ii. 204–5. The promise was made apparently in February 1708, confirmed in writing by the Queen, and accepted by Sarah in a letter of 31 Mar. The Queen was looking for a way out of the promise by February 1710 (Coxe, III. 52).

[108] Ibid. G-I-8 (Sarah's hand).

[109] Blenheim MSS. G-I-8 (fair copy). See diary entry for 16 Jan. 1711.

possibility that, since they could not be obtained by force, they might be returned via the Duke himself, other matters being satisfactory.

From the beginning of December until Sarah's dismissal, Hamilton was constantly the recipient of the Queen's orders and Sarah's letters. For example, Sarah, provoked by another issue of the *Examiner*, wrote lengthily to Hamilton on the 3rd 'to assure you I have all the Just esteem for you that you deserve & wou'd go a great way farther then London to serve you . . .'[110] The letter is endorsed in Sarah's hand that 'the q; let this man [Hamilton] read all these leters to her, & some times when she had not time, took them from him, & gave them again next time she saw him, but her way is to make little or no answer . . .'. Another letter came to Hamilton on the 5th which he relayed to the Queen, who dismissed it, and yet another from Windsor on the 6th. This is a long letter of justification and intended to reassure Hamilton regarding the printing. At the end of the letter she urges Hamilton

> to burn my letters, for in such a world as this they are not to be trusted with every body . . . I have an opinion that you are an honest man, & that you wou'd not betray me, tho our acquaintance was purely accidental, & I can see well enough your partiality for Mrs. Morley, at least you appear so, but as to that matter, I know tis impossible for you really to believe all you say upon her subject, after what you have seen & know to be true, but you are her servant, & I suppose she is kind to you, which is a very good reason for you to wish her well, & as long as I am call'd her servant which necessity has been the cause of, I do think the advice you have given me was right upon my own account as well as Mrs. Morleys . . .[111]

The Queen's only comment on 7 December was that 'The Duchess wrote free . . .'.

Sarah, perhaps feeling that time was running out, wrote again to Hamilton on the 8th mentioning his 'great businesse' and 'little leisure to read printed papers'. She went on to commend Marcus Antoninus '& his meditations' in order to set an example before the Queen of good government 'which is exactly the case of one that I know you love mightyly & therefore I wish you had courage enough to endeavour to doe her good, & to save her as much as you can from her base flatterers . . .'.[112] Hamilton apparently did not acquaint the Queen with this latest piece for on the 9th the Queen seemed finally resolved that 'she would never see her more, and it woud look odd to

[110] Ibid. (fair copy).

[111] Ibid. G-I-8. The letter is endorsed 'copy of a letter to 260 sent to ——' in Sarah's hand. Hamilton sent a copy of this letter to the Cowpers. A copy in Mary Cowper's hand exists (Panshanger MSS. D/EP F. 207).

[112] Blenheim MSS. G-I-8 (Sarah's hand).

keep her in, and she never come to her'. On the same day Sarah wrote to Hamilton, declaring her intention of coming to town on the 11th, 'since I am yet call'd the groom of the stole, & I have not order'd any thing for her, tho she is to have all things new at christmas . . .'. Sarah's letter is in response to Hamilton's short reply (presumably to her letter of the 8th) which wishes the Duchess were in town 'by which I see you are still Jealous that I have not a right conduct concerning Mrs. Morley, & the inclos'd paper for ought I know is the cause of it . . .'. She remarks, ironically, that

> if you are weary of my corespondence you may burn my letter before you read it, as I depend upon you to do afterwards . . . I will hope that you believe me your friend & that there is no need of giving me any new arguments upon Mrs. Morleys Subject . . . I long to see you or at least to hear if you have presented Mrs Morley with the meditations of the Emperor Marcus Antoninus, if you cou'd perswade Mrs. Morley to immetate him.[113]

On the 11th Hamilton was ordered to insist on the Duchess's not inflaming the Duke on his return. Predictably, Sarah reacted to Hamilton's visit with another letter:

> I have been wondering Ever Since I saw You, to find You so Earnest in perswading me, not to inflame, as you call it, my Ld M. at his coming Over, As if ye Qn Her Self, were realy desirous yt he shoud still Serve, tho' at ye same time she is prevail'd Upon, by Her Ministers, to give him perpetually such Mortifications as make it impossible for him to Serve, wth any Honour to himself . . .[114]

She has, she says, wanted the Duke to lay down for two or three years, which was also his wish, but he was at the same time desirous to conclude the war. The letter rehearses once more the humiliation of the Duke and herself. It concludes that 'wn I have more time I must write to you again upon Another Subject, for I cannot be easy till I have convinc'd You, yt I never was in ye wrong, in any thing to Mrs. Morley, & tho' you are very Partial, I am sure demonstration will convince You, & You shall have it as soon as my hurry of getting her things is Over . . .'. She again suggested the Queen read Antoninus in order to be instructed 'how to defend Her Self'. Hamilton must have been the hardest-worked royal physician of Anne's reign as he strove throughout December to placate Sarah, persuade her in certain directions, and keep the Queen from disquiet. On 12 December he was assured that the intention was to keep the Duke in if he 'would go into her Measures'. Yet the Queen feared the effect on Sarah of the various affronts offered to the Duke in Parliament at this stage for Hamilton was told to

[113] Ibid. (fair copy).

[114] Panshanger MSS. D/EP F. 207 (Mary Cowper's hand).

endeavour to keep Sarah from printing. It is surprising that Sarah did not immediately do so, for the pressure on the Marlboroughs increased through the month. Sarah wrote to Hamilton on 20 December, complaining that her enemies exploited the fact that she did not wait upon the Queen but instead sent messages to her. By doing so, they know that it 'will add to the uneasiness which they give the duke of Marlborough in all other things, their main poynt being to remove him from the Queen, & not to let him serve any more, the only thing in which I ever did or ever shall agree with them'.[115]

Sarah had in fact made one attempt to come to court in December, on the occasion of the Queen's coming out of mourning, which she did on Christmas Day. The *Conduct* notes it briefly thus: 'The same person, to try the Queen further, mentioned my coming to court, as what might be proper, on account of some *new clothes*, which, as groom of the stole, I had by her MAJESTY's order bought for her. But she presently charged him to advise me, as from himself, not to come.[116]

There are two other accounts, given by Sarah, one of which shows that the scheme as a means of getting Sarah to the Queen came from Hamilton. She notes in a letter that

> Just before lord marl: was expected in England, this friend of mine . . . came to me & perswaded me to goe to the queen to see her cloathes tryd on which I had broughte, which hee fancyd would succeed very well & disappoynt all the talk in the back stair against me . . . but upon his reading this leter to the queen, she charged him to hinder me from coming, but not to say that she did not allow it, which was in Effect to have me found fault for omiting what she would not let me do.[117]

Interestingly, this is a case of Hamilton taking positive action on his own account in order to try some form of reconciliation. Whatever Sarah tried at the end of 1710 was in no way calculated to bring her back into the Queen's favour but it does emerge from this that Hamilton on occasions told her more than the Queen commanded.

There was after this no chance of the inevitable being further delayed. Cowper noted on 22 December: 'Ds. of M. came to see me: untractable as to any Reconciliation with Q.; as also, by Sr. Dd. Ham., it appear'd the Q. is to her'.[118] On the 23rd Sarah wrote to Hamilton the long justification she had promised in her letter of 11 December. In a rare spirit of humility,

[115] Blenheim MSS. G-I-8 (fair copy) endorsed 'coppy to *260* . . .'. Mary Cowper took a copy of the letter (Panshanger MSS. D/EP F. 207).

[116] p. 264.

[117] Blenheim MSS. G-I-8 (Sarah's hand).

[118] Cowper, *Diary*, p. 51.

Sarah went through her service to the Queen and searched for the reasons of her being put out:

I have been very uneasy ever since I talk'd to you upon the subject of the queens having never given me any reasons for her change, because you seemd to goe away with an opinion that she must have don it, & indeed I can't blame you if you have that opinion, since I am confydent that there never was an instance before of any thing like what has happend in my case . . . & notwithstanding all your partiality to the q: you are too honest a man to differ with me in that poynt after I have made it out to you that she has not given me any such reasons, as you your self will say are good ones, that I hope to do entirely to your satisfaction without sending you such volumes as without retiring you could never read, & tho I did once shew you a great many papers in my own vindication when I was provoked beyond what human nature could bear, I am yet very tender of trusting out of my hands what must needs make any body melanchollу upon the qs Subject that wish her so well as I beleive you doe . . .[119]

The letter seems not be written with the thought of the Queen's reading it but more a direct explanation to Hamilton himself. The only possible reason Sarah can find is the Queen's accusation of 'inveteracy' against Abigail in October 1709. Hamilton is appealed to as an honest judge to accept the truth when he hears it. Hamilton was sufficiently convinced to beg the Queen on the 24th that Sarah be put out 'with Civility, least it shoud provoke her to print'.

The final stage of the quarrel was about to begin, for the Duke of Marlborough arrived in England on 26 December. On the 27th, the day before Marlborough was to see the Queen, she had a long conversation with Hamilton in which she reviewed the situation, over the course of the long association with the Duchess. Hamilton on his own initiative talked to Godolphin and the Duke about the crisis. He told the Queen that the Duke clearly wished to carry on, but equally important was to have Sarah *quiet* which he hoped for via Sarah's patience and the Queen's goodness. The year ended, ominously, with Sarah requesting the return of letters she had written to Hamilton from Windsor. The dismissal of the Duchess came eighteen days later, despite Hamilton's desperate attempts to effect a reconciliation (for a detailed account of 1–18 January, see Appendix A). On Hamilton's advice, the Duke carried with him to an interview with the Queen on 17 December a submissive letter from the Duchess, to be met by the Queen in an absolutely unyielding vein. The Duke returned with the gold key on the evening of the 18th.

[119] Blenheim MSS. G-I-8 (Sarah's hand). There is a copy in Mary Cowper's hand (Panshanger MSS. D/EP F. 207).

Hamilton's most onerous work for Queen Anne was virtually complete. There was occasional contact with Sarah after 18 January, which in the diary, goes up to 12 April, after which the Duchess is not mentioned in this particular context. The last extant contact between Sarah and Hamilton is a letter of Sarah's on 29 June 1711. It serves as a fitting conclusion:

I have had several times a mind to have troubled you with my letters, I shd be extream glad to be with you tho' but for one hour. my strength decays by ye Continual uneasiness I have in my Mind. I have a Continual drought & Inward heat, so yt if I had a little quiet I shd think ye Spa Waters might be good. I shd be oblig'd by knowing yr Opinion, & at ye same time pray acquaint me of ye Qns health, wch you know is, & ever shall be, of more concern to me yn my Own, wishing her all manner of happiness, in this world & ye next, & if I shd be so Unhappy as to end my days, in this Countrey, wch I fear is very likely, after my death do me ye Justice, as to Assure her, yt she has lost a very faithful servt. I am wth much truth Sr . . .[120]

After the Queen died, Hamilton sent his diary, as has been noted (see p. xvii), to the Cowpers for comments and advice. He sent with the diary other material including

an original Letter of the Duke of Marlborough's, which to serve Him, I read to the Queen, and Likewise some Originals and some Copies of the Dutchess of Marlborough's Letters, which I read to the Queen; and two Copies of the opinions of some Divines as to the Queen's Promise with Asseverations to the Dutchess, by frighting Her with which, the Queen complied to keep her in till the Duke came home, and to let her give up, instead of being put out, which was designed (so soon as my Lord Godolphin was out) with all the Marks of Dishonour that Mrs. Massam could prevail on Her Majesty to Show . . . My Lady Marlborough called back for some of Her Letters, and others which I copied are so writen, that none can read them but my Self, else I had sent more to divert Your Ladyp.[121]

The letter also summarizes clearly Hamilton's personal view of the matter, and, as always, indicates his concern for the Queen's health during the affair. Her medical condition was hardly improved by Sarah's actions.

Effectively Sarah did not function in her offices for most of 1710 and she clung tenaciously to her appointments until January of 1711. The erosion of her authority and credibility with the Queen reflects the steady erosion of the Whig control of ministerial office throughout the year. Sarah's decline is almost a paradigm of Whig fortunes in the months preceding the general election. Throughout this time the extraordinary figure

[120] Blenheim MSS. G-I-8 (Sarah's hand).

[121] Panshanger MSS. D/EP F. 200. Mary Cowper copied eight of Sarah's letters to Hamilton into the back of her copy of Hamilton's Diary.

of Hamilton is constantly to be glimpsed as intermediary, pacifier, giver of opinion, and general factotum. It seems to be the case that, if he were removed from the picture in 1710, the fortunes of the Duchess of Marlborough and the dubious peace of the Queen would have been very different from what they actually were. His shadowy quality is what renders him difficult to define for the historian. It was also what made him ideal for his role as servant to the Queen.

NOTE ON THE TEXT

THE text has been transcribed from Mary Cowper's copy (Panshanger MSS. D/EP F. 207, see p. xvii), which has been collated with her daughter's later copy (ibid. F. 229). There are a number of interpolations and marginal notes, occasionally in Mary's hand but more often in a different hand which seems to carry some authority in correcting. For example the manuscript (p. 21) reads under 4 December 1710: 'The Queen said they woud do well for the Dissenters'. This is altered by the corrector to 'that woud do well for the Duke', which, in the context, makes very much more sense. Similarly the following (MS., p. 34): 'and then my Lord Sunderland told him he knew the contrary to be false' is emended to '. . . contrary to be true' (13 Dec. 1711). Emendations, where they appear to be more logical, are absorbed into the text; otherwise they, together with the rare occasions when Lady Sarah's copy offers a different version, are noted at the foot of the page. Marginal notes such as 'Earl of Sunderland remov'd' (MS., p. 10; 15 June 1710) are incorporated into the text and noted.

NOTES

1. The custom of marking the transition from one year to the next on 25 March occurs in the diary only in the case of 1710 to 1711. Other transitions begin the new year at 1 January. The one exception has been altered to conform with modern practice. The span covered by an opened fold of the text is indicated at the head in italics. All date entries are followed by a full stop.

2. Contracted names, titles, places, and dates are silently expanded as are ampersands. Names indicated by letters around a dash are put in full.

3. Superior letters are brought down to the line.

4. Obsolete forms are replaced with modern equivalents. Thus 'ye' becomes 'the'; 'yn' becomes 'then'; 'yt' becomes 'that' etc. Long 'f' becomes 's', and 'll' becomes '£'.

5. Occasionally, elementary punctuation is silently introduced either as terminal punctuation or where the sense would otherwise be obscured. New sentences are given a capital letter.

6. Obvious errors are silently corrected e.g. '3st' to '31st'.

7. Spelling varies widely in the diary and no attempt has been made to regularize it.

8. Distinguishing between some upper and lower case letters is occasionally highly subjective and there is thus an arbitrary element in some editorial decisions. Generally where there is doubt, modern practice is followed.

9. Any other editorial alterations to the text are put within square brackets.

In the textual notes, '*M*' after a note indicates that it is Mary Cowper's hand, '*S*' Lady Sarah's, and '*X*' the unidentified emender to Mary's copy.

THE DIARY

The first translation of the gouty humour from the knee and the foot, first upon the Nerves and then upon the brain, was the imediate Cause of the Queens death, and disquiet occasion'd that translation. The translation plainly appears from the History of her Majestys complaints to her Death but in order to prove that Disquiet of Mind was the Cause of it, I shall shew that she had frequent returns of disquiet, and that they affected her by a gradual sinking of her Spirits and weak'ning of her nerves, till they were prepard to receive a translation of the Gouty humour upon them when a suitable occasion (such as a more than ordinary concern of mind) should happen to her.

Such Translations generally come suddenly because the preparatory sinking of Spirits, and weakness of the Nerves, passing under the unintelligible name of *Vapours* are too little regarded (especially if the Person looks now amiss in the face, as happens when the blood is Vitiated and from thence bad nourishment convey'd to the solid parts) till their weakness become at length so great, as to fit them for receiving such a fatal translation.

This Position I prove, first, from her Majesty's own authority in her exact account of the State of her health given to me in *May* 1703 In the following words, 'That within these seven years only she had been liable to Vapours with Faintness of Spirits whereas Naturaly it us'd to occasion Stool'. But this Ill effect did not continue, for the Cause ceas'd, and a succession of pleasures to her mind follow'd after the foremention'd disquiets, with which her spirits and mind were undoubtedly strengthned, and the Ill effects of her Grief sensibly remov'd, for then she was in a much better state of health than before, the death of the duke of Gloucester,[1] and the coldness between her Majesty, and her Royal Sister,[2] affected her with inward concern and her spirits with Sinking and faintness; so the pleasures which follow'd undoubtedly refresh'd her mind, and strengthned her Spirits, such as Success in forming an Union between *Scotland* and *England*, formerly attempted by her Predecessors, but in Vain;[3] her repeated Successes against the french king,[4] her Universal fame for Piety[5] both at home and abroad, which engag'd the love and confidence of all her subjects and the admiration of all Europe. With all which, it was impossible but her mind must be highly delighted. Who then cou'd have sully'd the Queens Character, and how glorious would her memory have been to all Posterity if at that time she had died.

But to this Pleasure of mind, and health of body there happend a Succession of disquiets, which by grieving her mind, made her less able to resist outward impressions, and importunitys, a Compliance with which, has loaded the latter part of her life, with Reflections, and now her Memory with reproaches; and by impayring her health, and weakning her Nerves, rendred them also less able to resist this last translation of the Gout, which was the cause of her Sudden Death. This brings me to give a Second *proof* that Uneasiness of Mind was the Cause of the translation of the Gout, by shewing from my personall knowledge, a succession of Disquiets that happen'd to her Majesty from the time of my first attendance on her, towards the latter end of the year 1708 to her Death.

I shall pass by the trouble which the Princes Death gave her, because the happiness of her marry'd State, and her inward concern of Mind, which follow'd his death are so well known.[6] As also the Estrangement between her Majesty and the Dutchess of Marlborough;[7] being able to say nothing of it, but from the Time her Majesty commanded me to wait upon her Grace, to convey her pleasure to the Dutchess and her answers to the Queen.

December, 1709. I'll begin therefore with an uneasiness which her Majesty appeared to have, about the beginning of December 1709.[8] The particular occasion I was not made acquainted with. But the seeing her inwardly affected, gave me an opportunity to Caution her against disquiets, and as her Phisitian, suggest the Ill consequences that might happen at that time from it. Her receiving this advice with so much Goodness, (I may say Thankfullness) convinc'd me how right my conjecture was. But

9th. visiting her the 9th. of that Month I was farther confirm'd therein, for entering the back Stairs I found my Lord Godolphin, then Lord High Treasurer, waiting till her Majesty came out of her Closet, and upon my comming in, he came to me to inquire for the Queens health (the first time of his doing so, and indeed his great gravity, passing with me as a forbidding Countenance, gave me no inclination to Converse with him).[9] I answerd 'that her Majesty was better of the Gout, that it had been more regular than usual, that she took nothing but spirit of *Millepedes*,[10] and that since the use of it she had taken fewer medecines than before'; to which he Replyd the oftner the boards are wash'd, the sooner they are impair'd.[11] Upon this Freedom of Conversation I told his Lordship that it was in his Power to prolong her Majestys life, by laying before her as few disquieting things as possible, but if there was an absolute necessity for it, to shun it at least at some certain seasons. Which he with wonderfull good nature,[12] and seeming pleasure undertook, adding, that if I would send him a line to inform him of every such season, he would do his utmost to keep her easy.

After his returning from the Queen, and my going in, I told her Majesty what had pass'd which She received exceeding kindly; thank'd me, and desir'd me to go on, and do according as he had appointed, only not to trouble too often least he should think it came from her.

22nd. The 22nd. her Majesty acquainted me that she knew I had been with my Lord Treasurer, because he had been with her, and told her, he was not come to discourse of any affairs with her, for if he had occasion to do it, he knew it was not a proper time.

23rd. And on the 23rd. repeated that he would not trouble her with any affairs till after Christmass, which shews how readilly he came in to keep her from disquiet and to act the part of a kind friend as well as a Minister of State.

24th. The 24th. he sent to me to give him in writing the times he was to omitt Business, at least disquieting business to her Majesty, vid the History. Then he express'd great pleasure in the prospect of keeping her Majesty quiet this way. His after care, and the success of it, prov'd that his words were not complimental, that Freedom from disquiets contributed exceedingly to her health, and consequently that disquiet must injure it. With concern he broke out, saying, You think I disquiet the Queen; what trouble can that give her Majesty for me to read a letter or two to her, or to make her walk to the Councill and hear her Lords discourse upon her affairs;[13] Its Uneasiness from Tattles that injures her most, and craving from her Majesty that which would not look so well for her to grant.

1710.

January 11th. The 11th. January following she told me that business would come on, and great pressing for Places,[14] and therefore commanded me to discourse my Lord Godolphin, which I did and he so manag'd it that when I visited the Queen on the 17th. she

17th. expressed her self exceedingly pleas'd with my Lords care to keep her Easy; Meeting him afterwards, I told him this on purpose to incourage the continuance of his care, as also what she said upon my pressing her to open every disquiet to his Lordship, viz that she needed not, he taking all the Care which it was possible for him to do, and also that if disquiets return'd frequently upon her Majesty it was impossible but that her health must suffer.

31st. On the 31st. she told me she was perfectly easy, and extremely pleasd with my Lord Godolphin's care of, not only as to his conduct mention'd, but as to his interposing his care to free her from disquiet upon my Lord Marlborough's absenting himself about a regiment the Queen wou'd have given to my Lady Massams brother Hill,[15] and upon a report of an address to her Majesty to remove my Lady Massam from her service.[16]

February 10. She told me she was under great Vexation, but such as my Lord Godolphin could not help her in, probably from her being secretly pressed to put him out, as well as my Lady Marlborough, which I am satisfy'd from her own words, and after actions she was most unwilling to do, and am of opinion, that what ever views others might have in getting out the Duchess of Marlborough as a method to dismiss my Lord Godolphin yet she had not.

11th. I mention'd to her what health she had from the keeping off, of disquiets by my Lord Godolphin, and acting for her at the time when occasions of disquiet met her, Yea the Menses happend to her as if she had been but 20 years old, the good effects of which care to ward off Disquiet I mention'd to her, to her death, on purpose to remind her not to be uneasy.

27th. Another succeeding occasion of Uneasiness happend in the affair of Dr. Sacheverel,[17] some insisting that he should be punishd more mildly and others that his punishment should be more severe.[18] Her own opinion she expressd to me, was, that there ought to be a punishment but a mild one, least the mobb appearing of his side,

March. shoud occasion great commotions and that his Impeachment had been better lett alone.[19] When she heard of the order in which the Mob mov'd, in pulling down the meeting-houses, each acting their proper part, some pulling down, others carrying away, and some burning, and all this so quickly as to be an argument, of its being dessign'd before hand,[20] she seem'd greatly concern'd, and this probably was the reason of her abovementioned Opinion, that the punishment shoud be mild, least the Mobb on his side shoud from thence take an occasion, to go on in their Disturbances, and to my Knowledge it was then proposed to her Majesty, that in her speech to the Parliament she should Comand her Bishops to reccomend to their Clergy, the Preaching against Vice, and not to meddle in Politicks, with which her Majesty seemd pleased, but how they remov'd the Impression, I know not. The same Person[21] acquainted the Queen, that if the difference of Party advanc'd higher, it would break in, upon all Relative Dutys, it being at that Pitch already, to produce differences between the most near Relations, so that by Progress of this all Practical Religion must be laid aside, and a bitterness of mind succeed, which might be followd with Revenge and all its Ill Effects. This made some Impression on her Majesty, for several times afterwards she ask'd me if the minds of people began to be more Easy.

31st. Seeing her Majesty disquieted I presum'd to ask if she pleasd to Command me to speak to my Lord Godolphin to which she Replyd that now he had so many things in his head, and that he was become as hot as the rest, and therefore desir'd I would not speak to him about her health. Which was a plain demonstration, of the success of outward endeavour to impress the Queen against him and that tho' there had been a great disquieting struggle between her own Inclinations, and the force of outward Pressure, yet she was a yeilding. For to my own personal knowledge, her natural calmness, was such, that a Continu'd Teazing as she termd it her self, woud make her yeild, unless she stood in the middle between the teazings of two different Sorts, and then her affection and Personal respect would cast the ballance between the two advisers, as is the common Temper of a good natural disposition.

April 4th. Her own words to me were, that if uneasiness would injure her, she had enough of That, now. My own Conjecture then was, that the Estrangement between the Queen and the Duchess of Marlborough, was come to that height (partly by her own absence from the Queen, partly by the endeavours of others to impress the Queen against her, and partly by her own letters to justify her self against all accusations) as made her willing, yea desirous to part with the Duchess[22] (my Lady Masham, being now more the object of her affection) but not that this should be a means of parting with my Lord Godolphin, for finding this to be the Consequence of it, unexpectedly to her, she was so extreamly concernd, that she commanded me to speak to my Lord Godolphin to influence the Duchess to make her submissions, and this very day upon my asking her Majesty, if she had seen the Duchess, since my mentioning that affair to my Lord Godolphin, she answerd, Once, and said 'twas to no purpose for him to speak to Her, and then committed the affair to me; with which also my Lord Godolphin seemd extreamly pleas'd, promising to write for the Duchess, who was then at Windsor, on purpose that I might speak to her. In

19th. the mean time Her Majesty told me she had made the Duke of Shrewsbury[23] with less trouble than she expected,[24] and now hop'd she should be easy, and to show her remaining inclinations to, and her good opinion of my Lord Godolphin and that what she said March the 31st. was from the suggestion of others. She then told me, that my Lord Godolphin woud not give her uneasiness unless they forc'd him to it and Visiting, My Lord Godolphin

20th. the 20th. at night, by her Majestys command, to know if my Lady Marlborough was come to town, he expressd himself thus, like a real friend (which I must declare I believe he was from his Conduct) as well as a faithfull Minister 'That he knew nothing of the Duke of Shrewsburrys comming in, that he believ'd it was owing, to the Queens Estrangement from the Duchess.[25] That the Queen seemd very Easie, which was a great Ease to him, that he should not give her any disquiet about the Duke of Shrewsbury and however the Queen pleasd to act, he would do his Duty, and as soon as the Duchess came to town I shoud see her'.[26]

21st. Acquainting her Majesty what had passd the night before, with my Lord Godolphin she seem'd extreamly pleasd with my design'd interview with the Duchess, but desir'd that before it happend, she might talk with me about it, an argument that her Majesty had not fully determind to part with the Duchess.

29th. Her Majesty asking if I had spoke to my Lord Godolphin, or heard from him any thing of the Duchess's being come to town, I answerd, that my Lord told me, that he had heard nothing of her these seven days.

May 10th. My Lord Godolphin acquainted me, that he had writt again, to my Lady Marlborough to bring her to town that I might speak with her.[27]

11th. The Queen told me that the Duchess made my Lord Marlborough, and my Lord Godolphin do any thing, and that when[a] my Lord Godolphin was ever so finally resolvd when with her Majesty, yet when he went to her, she impressd him to the Contrary. Whether her Majesty had this opinion, from her own observations, or from the Insinuations of others to shew her the neccessity of parting with both these, in Case of my Lady Marlborough's being dismiss'd, least after her dismission, by Governing them she might be at the Helm of all her affairs, and order as she pleas'd, I know not, but the latter I conjecture, from her present willingness to accept of the Duchess submissions, when before her desire was to have her out, upon whose removal they hop'd to obtain an Intire Change of the Ministry (the Bait with which they entangled the Queen to Change the Ministry). And also from her often Expressing her self thus, O that my Lord Godolphin would be parted from the Duchess of Marlborough I should be very happy. But the

15th. Her Majesty told me that she saw how concern'd I was for her quiet and health, and therefore desir'd me that I should not act any more with my Lady Marlborough, and that if just now she made her Submissions, it would give her but so much the more uneasiness which made me imagine, that upon the Queens discovering Relentings towards the Duchess rather than part with my Lord Godolphin, the pressing and teazing of her Majesty had been encreasd, and had succeeded. For at the same time she desir'd me to see, if it was possible, to bring my Lord Godolphin off from the Duchess; for that would be one of the happiest things imaginable. That she did believe the City would be in an Uproar,[28] if he was turn'd out, and she was perswaded that he greatly study'd her Ease.

16th. I acquainted her Majesty, that my Lord Godolphin said, it was impossible their Relation being so near,[29] and their Circumstances so united,[30] for him to break off, from the Duchess, but that there was nothing in his Power, he coud Act for her Service, but he woud do it.

19th. Going to my Lord Treasurer to repeat my desire of keeping the Queen Easy, he told me, that new changes would have Effects on the affairs abroad, either by retarding a good Peace, or forwarding

[a] when] (*M*) whenever (*M*)

a bad one,[31] and lay too great a weight on those who happen'd to be imploy'd in the Ministry and prove to the disparagement of the Queen abroad, and force her to turn back again.

22nd. I faithfully related what my Lord Godolphin said, and it pleases me in reflecting upon it, because it proved prophetical. I ask'd if it would not do her Majesty service to hear reason, on both Sides, and draw conclusions, from what was spoken with least of Party-heat, and By Ends; for said I, Madam, my Lord Godolphin has told me not only of your Majesty's good Memory, but Judgement, and that it was pity you did not trust it more. I askd at the same time, if it would be any service to her, or give her any quiet, if I got J.B.[32] to write letters to Holland, to know what is said upon that Side concerning any Changes already made, or talkd of, which she comply'd with.

June 6th. Her Majesty having inquir'd if I had seen my Lord Godolphin I acquainted her, as he desir'd, that his opinion was that the Preferment of Mrs. Masham should be her Majesty's Deed,[33] and not appear as a reward for doing service, Else it would be an Odium that she was in the party and so might be hated if her Preferment came after the Changes. I mention this as an argument of the greatest good nature.

15th. Earl of Sunderland remov'd.[b] [34] I acquainted her Majesty that I had seen the Duchess, that she had justified her Self, as being her faithful servant, and that her affection for her Majesty, made her, that she could not ſorbear endeavouring to keep her from hurting her self, when she saw that by the Influence of others her Majesty was in danger of it. That I condemn'd her for arguing by letter with the Queen,[35] that only serving to keep up the Estrangement. To which the Duchess said, it was hard to be deny'd that liberty, after the Possession of so many years affection, and intimacy, and when her Majesty's love was turnd from her by the insinuations of One, she had bred up, and plac'd about the Queen; and so Impress'd her Majesty concerning her, as to Create a Confidence in her Majesty towards her, that she had sav'd the Queen £80000, which her Sister Queen Mary, and other Princes had laid out.[36]

Visiting my Lord Godolphin that night he told me, that he found it was the Queens inclination, that it should be known that

[b] *Marginal note (M)*

she would make no other Changes, but my Lord Sunderlands;[37] which I coud Easily believe, because her Majesty her self orderd me, to say the same, viz that she would make no other Change, but not to disown the dissolution of the Parliament.[38] By which it appears not only that farther Changes were not her Inclinations, but that she did not know of them as in a Scheme,[39] but only by degrees as they fell out. This Vindicates her at least as yet from the aspersions of Insincerity she being brought to yeild to the Changes afterwards made, by the Sollicitations of those about her, contrary to her first design and Expectation. So that she might in Sincerity say no more changes would be, and yet upon changes happening, not be under any imputation. But while I vindicate her, I dare say nothing in favour of those who led her to do any thing that might sully her Character while alive, or her Memory now she is Dead. I have no positive Personal Knowledge who they were and what were theyr Steps, for I distinguish in this my account between what I know to be true, and what I only conjecture from that knowledge. My Business is only to Vindicate her that is gone.

16th. The Queen asking me what the people said, I told her, that from her making Sir Richard Onslow one of the Council,[40] they said it look'd as if she would keep a ballance now she had the affections of all her Subjects, and if she added some to allay the Heat of Others, a just Ballance might be preserved. That the fear of the City, was the loss of my Lord Godolphin, because he had been a great support to the Bank.

17th. Visiting my Lord Godolphin by a command from himself, he acquainted me that the Duchess of Marlborough woud wait upon me at my own house, which happend the 19th.

24th. The Queen asking the discourse of the City, I told her that their fear was Lord Godolphin's being out. A proof of which was their presuming to wait upon her, to beg that she would not change the Ministry, nor call a new Parliament they fearing that if a new one happen'd, it would destroy all that had been done by former Parliaments.[41] Mr. Eyles standing for Parliament-man, now upon the talk of the dissolution when before he could not be prevail'd upon;[42] and their Unwillingness to lend my Lord Treasurer £120000 any longer than for three months, the letter happening to come to him while I was there.[43] Upon which she answerd that she must trust the Providence of God.

July 3rd. Discoursing of my Lady Marlborough, she said, people took up a part of a Story, and their own imagination made it worse. Tho' she had not seen her, she suppos'd she was at the lodge.[44] I told her I heard that 200 Priests were come over.

July 8th. I acquainted her that my Lady Marlborough was come to town to which she said she believ'd so, because said she, when I went to town I saw a window open,[45] an argument that she was there. I said to her I imagin'd she woud not see you, 'till her Passion was over about my Lord Sunderland, for she was extreamly angry that her intercessions with your Majesty in so humble a manner were rejected. I added it is necessary that my Lady Marlboroughs being out be done in a way the least provoking. For a woman of Sense and Passion, provok'd, dos often turn Malicious, and that may force her to Print what has happen'd, for her own Justification. She says, its an argument of her patience, tho' so proud, and Passionate, yet to bear reflections as Guilty of disrespect to your Majesty and to have it said she carrys disrespectfully in not comming to Court, when my Lord Marlborough desir'd before his going out of town that she might have leave to stay away. The Queen said it was true, but that then, she shoud not come to St. James, and as to her printing her Justification, the Queen said, that when People are fond of one another, they say many things, however indifferent they would not desire the world to know.

10th. Visiting the Queen I acquainted her of my Lady Marlborough's Design to Print, and in it would be contayn'd what would reflect upon her Majestys Piety, such as breaches of Promise and Asseverations, and when a quarrell hapen'd between a Prince and a favorite, it was not like a quarrell between two private persons, but spread through all Countrays, and sully that reputation for Piety, Sense, and good nature, which her Majesty had every where so justly acquir'd. The Queen said, that she had made many Approaches to her in Vain. I said this might be remedy'd by not provoking her in the Method of dismissing her, by not putting her out by her self, till my Lord Marlboroughs Dismission, which to her would be much more acceptable, for the Duchess said that she took more pleasure in justifying herself, than your Majesty did in wearing your Crown, and that she wonderd that when your Majesty was so much in her Power, you should treat her so. The Queen said she would consider of it, commanding me to come to her the next morning at Eleven. I said I hopd from this she would be cautious of ever being too open to any future Favorite. Meeting with my Lord Godolphin he told me, that if the Queen would let the Duchess be easy, till my Lord Marlborough came home, then she might act in it as she pleases. But visiting the Queen next day, there was no opportunity for her Majesty to speak to me.

13th. The Queen had not determind as to my Lady Marlborough, nor yet the 14th.

15th. The Queen had been writing all day, and had not time to talk, but the 18th. order'd me to come every day 'till she had opportunity.

22nd. I advisd the Queen to be fully satisfy'd that they could advance money, least upon the Whigs refusal of it, a streight should happen, which would reflect upon her, and therefore she ought to make the Ministry positively assure her, that they could do it[c] that so she might not be blam'd for disregarding the Nations Credit; upon which she thank'd me, and said she would go upon very sure grounds.

24th. I acquainted her that it was said to be Mr. Wards[46] opinion, that the Tories could not answer the Funds, if the Bank would not, and that any who had any Friendship for her Majesty shoud make it their main study to keep her in the affections of the People.

25th. Visiting my Lord Godolphin He told me, that however they might say they coud advance money, yet either they could not, or must do it with great loss: for the Stocks being low,[47] in selling them at discount 10 or 12 p. Cent and lending their money for 6 per cent. they must be great losers and that People had not money in their Chests, but it was Credit upon such and such Measures taken, that made the Success of them and the Prospect of Peace from them so it is[d] the altering of such and such Measures, and not of this or that Person, or Parliament, that breaks credit.[48]

28th. Visiting the Queen, after going to read a letter from my Lady Marlborough, and she taking it herself to read, I repeated my Lord Godolphin's saying to her, that it was pity that Mrs. Massam had not preferment as her Majesty's own favour, because afterward it would pass as a Reward of her Acting for the new Ministry and so she would be hated; I had no acquaintance with her, but this was my Lord Godolphin's opinion.

[c] it] (*S*) *M's ms. torn* [d] is] (*M*) was not (*M*)

August 8th. Lord Godolphin put out.[49]

10th. Visiting the Queen and she asking me what was talk'd, I answer'd I always told her the putting out my Lord Godolphin would sink Credit,[50] more than the dissolution of the Parliament and that they talk'd of her Majestys Inclinations to the Pretender.[51]

11th. I set down from her own Mouth, what she said to the Commissioners of the Bank who came to suplicate her not to Change the Ministry nor dissolve the Parliament Viz. *I have no thoughts of making any further alterations.*[52] A reflection on those whoever they were, who advis'd her to give such an answer when they knew that by further pressing the Queen in the Progress of their Scheme, further Changes would happen, and so load the Character of the Queen with falshood, when she Spoke at the time as she really thought, their pressing of her being Gradual sometime before a particular change was to happen, and not at once to yeild to a whole Scheme. I Perswade my self, that however her indispositions, recurring faster upon her than heretofore, and her High opinion of, and confidence in those she trusted, might make her less[e] capable to look strictly into Matters, as they were represented, and so yeild up the management of every thing into their hands, in order to her less acquaintance with her own affairs, yet I am satisfy'd Her Piety would never suffer her to break her word, as she has been of late charg'd,[53] it proceeding from too much trust to others, and her Ignorance in her own affairs by means of this Trust, and her repeated indispositions. How willing are any of us, however alive in health, to give up the hearing of, or acting in affairs to a servant we intirely confide in, when at any time indispos'd, and if thus by self-reflection we consider'd her Majestys late Circumstances, we should not be so apt to load her with reproach. But our Corrupt Natures lead us to this Vice, and Party-heat has added strength to it, so that we are apt to shun all occasions of receiving true information, resolving to believe lyes, whereas if we put our selves always in the room, of the Person reproach'd, we should then be dispos'd to lessen the reproach cast upon others.

15th. I gave her the words by which was express'd the breaking of her word.

16th. I gave her the Queries[54] wherein was printed what I mention'd the

[e] less] (*X*) least (*M*)

day before, saying if Mr. Harley[55] would answer one of them her Majesty woud have no more to say.

18th. I saying I hop'd she needed not fear supply from the Bank to support Credit, she replyd, they only frighted people to put a stop to what was doing. I told her the dissenters did not stir as in Persecuting Reigns, because whatever Ministry came in, their dependance was on her Majestys Piety, good Natural Temper, and Promise. In Converse afterwards with the Duchess she mentiond to me how ungenerous it was to my Lord Godolphin who had been an old Nurse to her, and whom for so many years she had consulted as a Father, to send a Message of dismission, by the Duke of Sommersets[56] Coach man,[57] Mr. Harley and the Duke of Shrewsburry putting it on the Duke of Somerset as if he was the doer of it. For next day the Duke of Shrewsbury sent a Message to him telling him that he knew nothing of it, to which my Lord Godolphin answerd, that it woud have done him no harm to have known it. The Duchess also said that Mr. Harley would have kept still behind the Curtain, but the Duke of Shrewsbury finding the load to be too much upon him and that he needed some body in Council, forc'd Mr. Harley to appear, before which it was necessary that my Lord Godolphin as Treasurer shoud be out to make way for him.

23rd. The Queen telling me she had desird the Duchess not to come to her, orderd me to hear what she said, in obedience to which Visiting

24th.[f] the Duchess the 24th, she said that her stay from the Queen was not from disrespect, but with the Queens leave, given her by the Duke when he went to flanders, and also when the Duke took leave of the Queen he desir'd that the Duchess's places might be divided among her Children,[58] which she had promis'd, and seald with asseverations, but is not done. Saying also that Mr. Erle[59] let the Queen have a paper which she gave to the Duke of Somerset and he came to Mr. Erle with the Paper. This as a Caution not to trust the Queen, and that my Lord Marlborough had write to her, that the mortifications he received from his own Countrey were so many that could he take any pleasure, it would be in the great concern strangers had for him. That there was a heat raised, which would do mischief at home, and service to the French.[60] For her to pretend to be for Hanover,[61] when Harley impress'd her with all manner of Notions against that Familly.[62]

[f] 24th] *Marginal note (X)*

28th. Acquainting the Queen that my Lord Godolphin heard how she shoud say, that she wonder'd he did not go into the Countrey, she answerd she never said any such thing, but that he was too apt to believe what was said, which did him a mighty injury. I told her how readily the Duchess yeilded to go from Windsor to the Country when the Queen came to Windsor.

September 5th. I acquainted the Queen how Much the Clergys *Address* from the Countrey, was taken notice of,[63] and the Ministrys not answering the paper about breaking her word.

8th. I gave her Majesty *Querie upon Querie*,[64] telling her that my design in this, was, to keep up her own honnour by her imparting occurrences to her Ministry as well as they to her, and to save her from being impos'd upon, they not knowing, but if they did, this way a discovery might happen.

12th. I show'd her the *Bishops letter to his Diocese*,[65] still repeating that it would show the Ministry, that she was acquainted with more things, than what they imparted to her, and would make them fear to say any thing that was false, least it should be found out this way. I told her that Reasons were comming out, why the Bishops did not unite with the Address of the lower house, least they should be thought undutifull to the Queen.

13th. I show'd her the *Test of the Elections*.[66]

16th. The Queen ask'd me if I had heard any thing of the Duchess of Marlborough, because she had heard, she was in Town, and was a going out of it. I told her the Duchess had imparted to me a matter of great Secrecy, charging me to mention it to none but her Majesty, viz: that when she thought to have gone from the Queen she desir'd her Places to be given to her Children, which she promis'd, and that the Duchess sat down upon her knees, and desir'd a Solemn asseveration to seal it, which she granted. To which her Majesty answered that persons may Promise, and yet upon Occurrences change; To which I reply'd, that if in Friendship, to which my Nature much lead me, I made a Solemn Vow, albeit it[g] was to my prejudice I would be sure to keep it, according to that of *Psalm* 15, where its given as an Evidence, of a persons going to Heaven, *that he swears to his own hurt, and yet repents not.*

21st. I told the Queen how happy it would be if all her affairs were over, that she might go into the Countrey for Exercise, and for

[g] it] (X)

Ease to her mind, both which being of the highest consequence to her health, for it must needs be a great uneasiness to a person of so good a disposition as her Majesty, to put people out, when anger and rage were not the Motives, but supposed prudential reasons, and the Strong Sollicitations of those confided in, to which she answered, *And necessity too*, telling me that Mr. Boyles going out was his own doing.[67]

22nd. In discourse with her Majesty, that since the dissolution of the Parliament the night before, people would now know what to expect, and would be easier. She saying on my showing her *Now or Never*,[68] that Dr. Clark[69] was a good man, and upon shewing her the *letter to the Examiner*[70] and *the Essay upon Credit*,[71] she said the Author was not *D'Avenant*[72] but tho' she knew him, yet must not discover him;[73] and that *Sacheverel* was a foolish man, for going into the Countrey.[74]

23rd. I told her that Two things griev'd the Clergy and made them afraid of the Pretender. One was, that of Mr. Hoadleys[75] Account of the Marquis of *Carmarthen's*[76] saying, that he was to go to bring over the Prince of *Wales* to which she said, That no such thing was under his Hand: that it was spoke when He was drunk, and in the Night to his Mistress.[77] Another was the Story of the Jacobites from Scotland, offering to come in if she would compromise and let the Pretender succeed her. Comming out from the Queen I met the Present Lord Chancellour Cowper,[78] going to give up the Seals, with whom I went home to his House, and press'd his staying in, by Order from the Queen, She Refusing that day to take the Seals from him.[79] To which he answer'd;[80] That the honour and Emmoluments of such a place were not to be despisd, yet to Enjoy them in such a way as he must, he could never think of; That tho' by his Place he was principally to be advis'd with in Dissolutions yet all this to be done, for them to carry to him, as if he was not worthy to be advis'd with, was what could not well be born: that[h] *Mr.* Harley not expecting to see him at Council,[81] upon Sight of him, about a quarter of an hour before it sat, went in to the Queen, and told her it was not fitt my Lord Cowper should be surpris'd with the dissolution. Whereupon the Queen call'd him in, and said she had resolv'd upon the Dissolution, to which he said, then it was to no purpose for him to say any thing against

[h] that] (*X*)

it, and when the Council met, the Queen askd if the Proclamation was ready. The Attorney General, now Lord Harcourt,[82] Immediately took it out of his pocket, and in a Minute the Clerk[83] had read almost the half of it, (which was a Sign he had practic'd it before). When it was read the Queen imediatly withdrew, and would not hear any person Speak; which was not right; Tho' Speaking could not hinder her determination yet by Oath he was oblig'd to Advise, Silence giving a Consent, so that it may be thought it was done with the advice of the Privy Council, but it was not, for she would not suffer them to speak, and what will not bear debate, ought never to be advis'd, no more than what will not bear the light. There were words in the Proclamation it self to be debated expressing the Motive to it, which were wrong, viz: the Addresses which reflected on so great a part of her Nobility and Gentry.[84] I cant keep in, unless I go to such a height, as would give the greatest uneasiness in my Own mind. For they carry on things, by Trick and Contradiction and Shuffle, which will make the Queen lose her honnour and the affection of her People. I remember likewise, by order of the Queen pressing further the Chancellour to stay in he said to this Effect, that his respect was great for the Queen. He never as he believ'd, displeasd her in any thing but this. He never bore on her to Determine a thing, against her mind, which was the fault of some, and one of his arguments for laying down, was to serve her, for by keeping up a reputation with the rest, he would be able to serve her, if the way she was in did not do. This was a Practice Honourable in him, kind to the Queen, and what has succeeded before, as in *Strada* the Jesuites, History of the Wars in Flanders,[85] when measures are taken, which almost Universally disoblige one considerable part of the Kingdom, there is no way so likely to serve the Princes, in Case the present measures shoud fail, as by preserving a Reputation with those, who think themselves injur'd. It was an Argument Us'd by the Nobility of Flanders to *Margaret*,[86] when oppress'd by the Ministry of Cardinal Granvile[87] who had her favour at that time, as Mr. *Harley* has the Queens. And it had its Effect, for he so inflam'd the Kingdom, that had it not been for them they had been Undone and She too.[88] The Lord Chancellor brought the Seal again the next day and deliver'd it up,[89] and other Changes succeeded.[90]

24th. I told her Majesty that I had spoke to my Lord Cowper, with how much respect he spoke of her, but that he could not keep in. It would appear like Coveteousness in him. Besides he could not join with them for he saw nothing but Trick and Shuffling. He that should have had the main hand to know nothing, and by His Oath should have given Advice not to be heard, bore hard upon him; To which she said *That there was a precedent for what she did.* I told her she was reflected upon, as if she had broke her word, begging she would be cautious of being made to promise any thing, which she was not certain was in her Power to fullfill, because I knew her Sincere Piety, which Evil Persons by such a handle would be apt to reflect upon. I had heard her Majesty reflected upon by some of the Clergy for not sending for *Doctor Bradford*[91] as She promis'd. I told her also I had excus'd it from her Multitude of Business. She told me she had promis'd it and designd it, but had forgot it. She order'd me to tell my Lord Cowper he shoud come now and then to see her.

27th. Her Majesty being to go to Windsor, commanded me to write to her, and take care it came safe to her hands; asking at the same time if my Lady Marlborough were in Town, desiring me to get notice in order to acquaint her, the next day.

28th. The Parliament was dissolv'd the 21st.[1] I told her that neither my Lord Godolphin nor the Duchess were in Town. She repeated her commands, that I shoud take care in writing not to sign my name.

October 7th. Waiting upon Mr. Harley about a Person in Distress, whom I had introduc'd to the Queen before the Change of Ministry.[92] In Converse about Lord Cowper He said his going out was concerted, and that he had dipp'd himself, so farr, by promise to the others, that he could not go off.[93] I said it was Pity, because he Valu'd the Queen and was Sincere, and I mentioning Dr. Bradfords case to him, he said his hinderance was Standing on his own terms. In commending the Queens Integrity, I told him People said he would learn the Queen to Equivocate.

10th. Visiting the Queen at Windsor, I told her I had been with Mr. Harley, and told him some people said, he would learn her Majesty to Equivocate, as also with how much good nature he received it. I hop'd he was not what the world thought him to be, but Sincere,

[1] *Marginal note (M)*

To which she said she hop'd so, and told me she had heard of the letter to the Freeholders.[94]

16th. Visiting the Queen I mention'd only the bill of Comprehensions,[95] wishing she would begin it.

30th. Shewing her my Lady Marlborough's letter, she told me that she wrote free; and that the Earl of Rivers was barbarously treated at *Hanover*.[96] I said that the Duchess told me that matters were so now, that it must be the Prince of Wales or Prince of Hanover.

November 8th. The Queen unwilling to hear of any thing about the Duchess.

29th. I show'd a letter of the Duchess of Marlboroughs to her.

30th. The Queen discoursing of having her Original Letters from the Duchess of Marlborough, in order to make what she said of less Value, for if that was seen or printed, *That she wish'd never to see heaven, if ever she parted from her*,[97] how reflecting that would be. And since the letters coud not be taken away by force, perhaps upon my Lords comming over matters might be so settled, as that she might have them. The *Queen said all these promises were nothing now*. I said she knew that best, but that I durst not say so, and would endeavour if possible, to obtain them from the Duchess, because I found her extremly willing to gratify her Majesty in many things. And my Influence seem'd to be a Reward for my Integrity both to the Queen and to the Duchess, I having no by End, but her Majesty's honour, health and quiet of Mind.

December 1st. She Returnd the Duchess's letter, telling me how good natur'd the Duke us'd to be, that he could not give any Creature a harsh word; whereas lately he appears so illnatur'd, and swearing, that he could not forbear swearing in her Presence.

4th. Reading my letter to the Duchess, to the Queen, she commanded me to keep a Copy; I told her that she would be a continual thorn in her Side, if care was not taken to carry with as little provocation as possible; and that according to her Commands I woud endeavour to keep her from meeting the Duke.[98] The Queen said that woud do well for the Duke.[j]

5th. I show'd her the Duchess's letter, to which she said, Her passionate temper made her receive ill impressions before she knew the truth of a thing; And upon my mentioning the imputation upon my

[j] that] (*X*) they (*M*); Duke] (*X*) Dissenters (*M*)

Lord Treasurer as to the Navy Bills,[99] O fy, says she, its rather upon my Lord Churchill.[100]

7th. The Duchess wrote free, the Duke of Sommerset never told a lie of her, and that my Influence upon her seem'd to be a reward for my integrity.

9th. The Queen was then positive she would never see her more, and it woud look odd to keep her in, and she never come to her.

11th. The Queen order'd me to insist that she might not inflame the Duke. She hopd my Lord Marlborough would be calm, and submissive. I promised my utmost endeavour, telling the Queen that my design was to keep her Majesty from being provok'd, and the Duchess from being despis'd.

12th. She told me, that they went up and down the Army, making factious Officers,[101] that would be put out, and shoud have the money, but she woud state the Price.[102] And asking the Queen if she design'd the Duke shoud serve, She answerd *to be sure, if he would go into her* Measures, and not divide and make partys; and desir'd that I would endeavour that the Duchess shoud not print.

13th. She commanded me to tell the Duke and Duchess that this was not done with the least disrespect to the Duke; but because they had made it their Business to reflect upon her, and her administration, therefore she would do this that it might be an Example to Others.

14th. Reading what pass'd between the Duchess and I, she said Cadogan[103] was a sad fellow.

15th. She told me she had done something, at which she believ'd the Duchess would be angry Viz, made Lord Hertford Governour of Tinmouth.[104] That the Duchess of Somerset[105] was no liar, but might say passionate things, tho', never to her. Telling the Queen that the Duchess said he would not go to Council, and that she wish'd he might be put out. To which the Queen answered, She'll be mistaken. I told the Queen how kindly my Lord Godolphin spoke of her, and even of Mr. Harley, too; is that says she since he was out, to which I said, Yes, and that if her Majesty did not take it amiss it was kind to go to him now he was out, I having had Experience of his Care to keep her from Disquiet. To which she said, Yes by all means, as also, that my Lord Marlborough would begin with her.

16th. She express'd her thoughts as if my Lord Marlborough would not comply with any thing, etc.

19th. The Queen ask'd if the Duchess said any thing of the Duchess of Somerset. To which I answered That I had always heard that the Queen had a respect for her, and that by reason of her Quality and disposition she seem'd suitable for Her; and I hop'd she would be carry'd through the doing it[k] without disquiet to her.

24th. Visiting the Queen she told me that the intire defeat in Spain was true;[106] and begging that the Duchess might be put out with Civility, least it shoud provoke her to print.

26th. I having been at Rochester acquainted the Queen, of the Evil of Party, because it made the Clergy preach on that, instead of practical Religion, and made the people go beyond all tyes of Relation, and friendship, telling her what happend when I was there, That it was only in her Power to keep a ballance, and so long as such pernicious Sinfull Heat was kept up, more judicial Punishments besides the loss of Spain woud happen; however a Religious Example, she gave her self; telling of the Nonsensical Distinction of Tory and Whig in Heads, and giving her that Excellent Sermon of Dr. Bradfords, on that Text; the Wisdom which is from above is first pure, peaceable etc.[107]

27th. The Queen told me that the putting out of Wright,[108] and putting in Cowper, made no difference between the Duchess and her, for the Duchess had never spoke but once to her of it;[109] and once of Lord Sommers,[110] saying it was Mrs. Masham who hinder'd it, when She knew nothing of it, nor did not know him. The Duchess never spoke to her of Lord Orford,[111] but if in printing all this be said, it makes her mightilly in favour with the other Side, and as for the Duchess saying, that the Queen said she was not chang'd, No more she said she was, for she had never said any such thing Since her heart was turnd from her. I then said that the Duchess's Carriage from fear, and suspition of Mrs. Massam turn'd your Majesty the sooner to Mrs. Massam, who carry'd at that time in a more acceptable way to you. That the Duchess had said shocking things Even to her self, Yea as much to her self, and afterwards in Company,[112] as that she lied. And as to that promise the Duchess mentions, she had not behav'd her self suitably to it, and so it was null. To which I said if there were no asseverations, she Reply'd,

[k] it] (*X*)

I believe not, because tho' one in the heat of affection and expression from thence might say many things, which they would not in writing, besides that was not her way, neither did she assevere as to the Children, for they deserve so little; The one is cunning and dangerous to be in the Familly,[113] the other Silly and Imprudent, and lost her Reputation,[114] and Montague was just like her Mother[115] (One would not say this to them). Besides I have put out her husband[116] and that wont look well to have her have Her Places. The Duke said indeed that his Wife was for having it put into execution, but he had prevail'd upon her, not to think any more of it now; and that the Queen said to put it by, that it would not be so well now. I said if it was in half a year, that needed not alter the Resolution of putting her out. Besides she said she would never Meddle in any thing. Is her promise therefore to be depended upon, saying that the Duchess wrote to me as she us'd to do to her. I said my Lord Godolphin was for the Dukes Serving, but the Queen said the rest would irritate him, and the Duchess would provoke him, but theres more hopes if Godolphin be for it. And to Shew the Queens respect to my Lord Godolphin and Dependance upon his Opinion, she desir'd me to go to him, to have his Opinion, what Method to take as to the Affair in Spain, which he did in Writing as follows, vid. the letter.[117]

29th. She told me my Lord Marlborough had been very humble, and submissive last night,[118] and Visiting Lord Godolphin he told me that my Lord Marlborough had carry'd Mildly, assuring the Queen that he would serve her as long as he coud do her any Service, and that it was not a time now to take notice of any Mortifications given him. Then visiting Lord Marlborough he told me he had assur'd her, he would serve her, tho' the Warr was now more difficult abroad by the Turks coming into the North, by sending Men to Spain, by the French being strong in Italy, Germany, and the low Countries.[119] If he stayd at Home, the Unsuccessfullness would be imputed to his not being there. All which prov'd, that his service is meer Duty and Submission to the Queen. That he would not intrigue with any Ministry, but do them all the Service he coud, in the State of the Warr; That his great Uneasiness was to have her made Easy, which he hopd, by her having more Patience, and the Queen more Goodness might be done.

30th. Visiting the Queen I faithfully related what pass'd with the

Duke of Marlborough, how affectionately he Spoke of her, which melted her, That he said that he long'd to have his Wife quiet,[120] which nothing could do but the Queens goodness, and her Patience, as said above, that it was Duty and Submission to the Queen that made him serve now. At this time it was more difficult, because the War was in a worse posture, and he would have more difficultys, for he did 20 things before, which he could not, Yea durst not do now, but depending on the Queens Favour he would not lay down. I said to the Queen he needed to have his mind easy by Smiles, from her self. The Duchess told me that if the Queen smil'd or said any thing pleasant he thinks nothing amiss. Her Majesty said she was sorry to see him so broken. That there was no thought of putting him out.

31st. Received a letter from the Duchess desiring her letters which she had wrote from Windsor to me, which the Queen saw.

1711.

January 1st. Being with the Duke and Duchess she told me of Argyles[121] not having money to pay for his Instalment, wherby it was stop'd, as also Mr. St. Johns[122] telling the Queen of the Dukes going to Montague house and of Granvile's[123] Secretary of War, his calling at my Lord Marlborough's when he knew he was out, and then sent his man to do business with the Duke. The Duke also said that if Mr. Harley and Mrs. Massam were not willing he should serve, they might make him incapable of serving by refusing Supplys.

2nd. Visiting the Queen I told her that the Duchess said, that it would be both generous and Christian for her to say to my Lord Marlborough, bring Lady Marlborough with you, and when she comes to say to her, I pass by what has been amiss on condition you carry your Self right for the future. To which the Queen answered, I have said that to her before; to which I reply'd that I had heard the Duchess say after her last letter, that she would meddle neither with Politicks, nor with Mrs. Massam. Her Majesty also said that the Duke look'd better, and that it was only Fatigue. When the Queen first saw him, and me soon after, she took notice of his looks with concern, and from her self believ'd it the effect of Disquiet but others vex'd to see this good inclination in the Queen Nois'd that in her Ears, that it was only Fatigue;[124] Every one knows how impressive a Conversation is, when it is constant, and the Person lik'd with whom it is. I say this to show the natural good inclinations in Her Majesty's self, however kept dormant and Clouded and misrepresented, from the Impressions of others.

5th. The Queen told me that the Duchess in her letter said that her Majesty did, and said so, but never own'd her self doing or saying so; To which I answered that Self Vindication was natural, and so fixing the mind to it, that when they were about it, they seldom thought upon Self accusation, they seeming Contradictory. Its generally a Spirit of Religion, or great Generosity that Unites them together at one time. The Queen also said the Reason why she desir'd the Duchess to write without coming to her was, because one can write ones thoughts as well as say them, especially its better in her, because when she speak them it is always in Passion, which is uneasie to me. The Queen also said that the Duchess said, that what she had to say needed no answer, and therefore the Queen took hold of her words, and so gave no answer.[125] The Queen also told me, that when the Duchess left her, she said, that God would punish her either in this world, or in the next for what she had done to her this day. The Queen said that it was very hard passing a Sentence upon any body, for that was a thing, between God and themselves, and yet said the Queen that was no shocking thing according to her, for she says that she says no shocking things to me, but that I say them all to her. The Winter after the Prince dy'd, there was a Closet which the Queen Mother[126] had made for the Priests to come to her, which she said I us'd to be in, with Mrs. Massam some hours, when I was there on Melancholly Occasions.[127] To which I said, That Suspition was the Effect of her fear of losing your Majesty's affection, and of its fixing on Mrs. Massam.

The same day at night my advice was received by the Duke and Lord Godolphin.

6th. Visiting the Queen I told her how angry my Lord Duke was to hear that the Duchess shoud have spoke so to her Majesty, with which she was extreamly pleas'd.

Visiting the Duke at night, I prevail'd with him to talk and carry affectionately as a suitable preparatory help to obtain what there's some hopes of Viz her Majestys forgiveness upon the Duchess's owning her Faults by letter.

8th. Visiting the Queen and telling her however the Duchess was passionate, yet I was satisfyd of *His* tenderness and affection toward her Majesty, she saying what Passion the Duchess sometimes would be in, and how she would keep her in till it was over. The Queen also told me, Mr. Harley would be easy with the Duke, and that it would be no more disgrace to him to have the Duchess out than in.[128] To which I said that his concern was least the noise of it abroad shoud lessen him, as if he was not so much in the Queens favour, and so he be less capable to serve her. For it was by the Character of the Queens favour to him, that he was so successfull, they from thence trusting his Promise, as if it had been her Majesty's own.

10th. Visiting the Queen I told her of an Oath by which she had bound her self to the Duchess. To which the Queen said that there was no Precedent of the Duchess and that her Oath was conditional on her behaviour. To which I said I would go a great distance to have her letters to the Duchess up, it would so disparage her Majesty to have them printed. Might not a Reconciliation betwixt the Duke and Mr. Harley forward a forgiveness to the Duchess, but she said it could not be done. Then Visiting the Duke and Duchess, and discoursing what happen'd, the Duchess said, Give me a reason or a Precedent where a Mans service has been regarded as Useful to the Queen and Nation, and his Wife put out of her Place, in which she had serv'd faithfully for 27 years. I dont know what Counsels the Queen has, but theres nothing like this in Turky, in Neros time, or in any History. I know its so impossible for my Lord to submit to it, that I earnestly desire, to know of the Queen, if she be not in the Secret with the Ministry, who have contriv'd this way to make him quitt; not daring to turn him out, because its so unpopular a thing. Then she told me of two parts of a letter, or letters she had from the Queen, one, *I wish I may never see the face of Heaven if ever I consent to part with you.*[129] Upon which the Duchess said; How can a Religious Person, be easy in their own Mind in putting out a woman in such a manner, even tho' she committed a fault, after such an Oath written and seal'd under her own hand. Another part *I wish I may never enjoy happiness in this world or the next, for Christ Jesus's sake do not leave me.*[130] These two, I own, were writ at a time when the Queen had a kindness for me, and now I have the misfortune to be under her displeasure, but still it makes no alteration to attend her Conference between God and her self. And whatever the Queens Passion and my Ennemys may occasion at this time, if she reflect upon this it must trouble her when she comes to die. The Queen cannot help not loving me but she can keep from abusing me. Such Things are in my Power, that if known by a Man, that would apprehend, and was a right Polititian might lose a Crown. But I shall do nothing against her which I would not have done 20 years a go, unless Provok'd. I us'd to tell her of every ones faults, however so near to me, and even of Mr. Churchills,[131] on which she wrote to me, *he has not all the good Qualitys which are to be desir'd, but if people were not so full of Malice and Passion, as to turn their heads, they would not be so uneasy to a Man thats so near the Duke of Marlborough.* Vid. the handsomness of that Stile, Its Easy to her to spare an ill man because of his Relation to the Duke, and at the same time spares not his wife, who has done no Ill thing and is nearer to the Duke of Marlborough.

My Own Scheme for Reconciliation in Order to keep the Queen Easy, but it did not extend far enough to supplant what was to follow. (1st) by reconciling my Lord Marlborough and Mr. Harley, by which the Duke would Impress the Allies abroad with a Confidence in Mr. Harley, and Credit would at the same time rise at home. (2ndly) between the Queen and the Duchess of Marlborough, by the Duchess's first submission by letter, next the Dukes intercession and then her own personal submission, The Duchess being willing never to mention the least thing displeasing to the Queen, by which her Majesty would be kept quiet. (3rdly) between the Duchess and Mrs. Massam, the former yeilding to the Queen's doing Favour to the latter, Now by this means Mrs. Massam is the Favorite and Mr. Harley the Minister, and yet the Queen kept quiet.

12th. I was at some pains to read the Annotations on the 15th Psalm, and on Ezekiel about an Oath,[132] in order to convince the Queen of the danger of breaking it, and Visiting her afterwards she told me, that there were various circumstances which lessen'd the Oath, such as, the time of it, when she was at Variance with her Sister Queen Mary, and her undutifull behaviour since.

13th. Visiting the Queen she told me, that the late King William put my Lord Marlborough in the Tower, for things which were falsly alledg'd against him.[133] And upon the then Princess's going to

Queen Mary, to see her, Lady Marlborough being in waiting went with her, but the Queen took no notice of her, upon which, she knew something was a coming, and then the Queen writt that she shoud put out Lady Marlborough.[134] Messages went between Queen Mary, and the Princess Anne for some days, then the Princess went to the Duke of Sommersets, and it was at that time she wrote that letter to the Duchess of Marlborough.[135] The Queen also told me, the last time the Duchess was at Kensignton, she came back again, and said to her, she hop'd she would not affront her openly; Upon which the Queen said she never did that, in her life, to any, and that to be sure she would not if my Lord Marlborough express'd himself well, and thereby insinuated himself with them, who could do him service, he would stay in, for he's Ambitious and wont go out. In comparing this, with the Queen's fear of his going out, its plain that this Expression, was from outward Impression, and the fear from her self, and her Own Inclinations to him. She told me she was easy in that promise, as to Her self, saying, If the Duchess offerd to kill me, must not I put her away; and dos she not go about to take away my Name and Reputation, which is all one. She had not yet consider'd that Affair, but told what Bishop —— said vid. a Bishops opinion of that promissory Oath.[136]

15th. Her Majesty told me it was known the Duchess wrote to her, and that I had seen the letters, and ask'd if ever I said so my self, to which I said No. I gave the Duchess's letter to her, and discours'd about the Duchess's staying in, till the Duke went out also, To which she reply'd How can that be for her to keep three Places, and not attend. I read the Bishop's Opinion, and gave her in, another Divines which I had taken in writing.

16th. Visiting the Queen she told me that the Duchess said to her in Passion, that she wish'd the Queen might be in difficulty, and in Her Power, only, to help her, that she might have the Pleasure not to do it. Desiring that she should be put of that of talking with a Minister, and that her proposal of staying in till my Lord went out, was impossible, ordering me not to challenge her, for saying, that I read her letters to the Queen, for fear of falling into a Flame.

17th. Visiting the Queen, she order'd me, that if they spoke of her laying down, to give in to it, but not to mention it, either to him, or her, as of my self; the Queen saying that if my Lord cry'd a little it would then be over; I mention'd how ill he was, and how affected, and said, that his dependance was on the Queen's Compassion for him.

18th. Visiting the Queen she told me the Duke had been there,[137] and was not so tender as one might have expected; and said it would be more for his, and her quiet, to prevail with her to Lay down; he said he would endeavour it; and if in a forthnight he could not accomplish it, she might do what she thought best; and this being concerted, order'd me not to go unless they wrote, To fulfill which Promise, I wrote an Excuse to the Duchess for not coming.

19th. The Queen told me, the Duke had brought the Key last night.[138]

20th. Visiting my Lord Cowper, he told me that when some Lords told the Queen that they would Vote for the Interest of the Nation, she bid them vote as the Lord Chamberlain[139] did, That the Queen's known Favour for the Duke, was one great occasion of his Success. For at the battle of Ramillys, the Danes unwilling to fight standing upon their Arrears, and their dependance upon it, as if it had been from the Queen, made them join, and was suppos'd to contribute greatly to the Victory of that day. That the Scheme Lords,[140] the Neccessitous Lords,[141] and the Scots Lords[142] Vote according to the Ministry, but the wise and Independent Vote, according to Judgement.[143]

22nd. Visiting the Queen, she told me the Duke was not Generallissimo.[144] I read the Opinion of a Divine, she was pleas'd I should consult, about the Promise. I advising her, for the future not to make a promise, without expressing the Condition, not to say any thing to a Favorite, which would injure Her, if it came to be known. By this she would be free from all Tyes, and in no bodys Power. I said that it was expected some after favour, should be shown to my Lord Marlborough (1st) to prevent the Surmises that the Ministry will not suffer him to continue, (2ndly) That he may have the more Honour, and Credit, abroad; and so be capable to do the more service for your Majesty.

24th. Vid. the inconveniency of Putting in the Duchess of Shrewsburry.[145]

29th. The Queen telling me that my Lord delaware[146] ask'd how he should Vote, and she said, according as the rest of the Ministers.[147] I told her, I remember'd with great Pleasure, how she answered, my asking, for Mr. Stewart[148] from Scotland, how he should Vote; Viz According to his own Judgement, and had told it greatly to her Reputation.

February 1st. Visiting the Queen, I told her, I was to see the Duchess, she orderd me to endeavour to keep her silent, and not to expose things; not to stay too long, nor begin with her.

2nd. Visiting the Queen I gave her the Duchess's letter, telling her it was necessary to see her, that she might not take notice of me; for she had mention'd to Lady Cowper[149] that she did not know, but that I might read a letter now, and then, to the Queen. Other People might suspect me also, and frown on me for it, For tho' I need not matter their Frowns yet it was better to be without them.

9th. The Queen orderd I shoud not go to the Duchess of Marlborough till she sent.

12th. I mention'd how the Pious part of the People were pleas'd with taking the Convocation off from Hereditary Right, and Passive Obedience, to fix their thoughts against Immorality and Atheism, hoping this would strengthen the endeavours after Reformation.[150] To which the Queen said, that would be very well.

15th. Visiting the Queen, I let her know what pass'd with the Duke and Duchess in discourse. That the Duchess said, it had been kind if the Queen had waited 'till after the Campain, and then both of them to have laid down together; and so have Visited the Queen Civily in 3, or 6 Months. I told her also, that the Duke ask'd me what People said, of his Conduct towards the Queen and Nation, and that I told him, some gave him as Great, or greater Character, for that Victory over himself under the Provocations, than for all his other Victories; to which he said he would do his utmost, to maintain her Honour abroad, and that if there was a battle there might be a Peace; and desir'd me to Visit the Duchess, that when he was gone, she might not say, or do, anything to Provoke the Queen. He hop'd for his sake the Queen would be kind to the Children, whatever faults the Mother was guilty of and promis'd to write to me.

March. In this Month the Queen's Feavour, took away the opportunity of Converse.[151]

22nd. I told the Queen my Lady Marlborough ask'd for her, and said she had more relentings towards her, than she had this Six Years.

24th. Her Majesty discours'd, of the Duchess's Affectionateness, and not being inrag'd, and of the Dukes Prudence.

26th. Endeavouring to impress the Queen well, as to Lady Sunderland.[152]

April 9th. The Queen told me of my Lady Sunderlands informing her Majesty of the Duchess's asking for her by me, which she had a great sence of.

12th. Discours'd about my Lady Sunderland, she giving leave I should go to my Lady Marlborough.

18th. Discoursing how the Duchess own'd that in the Summer she advis'd the Duke to lay down.

May 5th. I was taken ill.

31st. The Queen told me she believed Mr. Harley (now Earl of Oxford)[153] was an honest Man.

June 26th. The Queen in discourse with me, told me Dr. Ratcliffe[154] was the last man she would take in, and gave me leave to say so.

August 3rd. She mention'd what Dr. Mead[155] said, he mov'd for Steel,[156] but she did not go into it. And that he said one thing she never heard before, that the Bath was not proper for the Gout.

27th. I went to the Bath, but being Ill was not able to say as much as I designd.

September 28th. Visiting the Queen in Return from the Bath, little Conversation.

October 12th. The Queen Speaking of my Endeavour to bear up her Reputation.

November 28th. Mentioning the Bishop of Salisbury saying, We are ripening for Judgement, and that the Dutch come into the Peace by Force.[157]

29th. Visiting Her, I let her know the Rage my Lord Cowper was in at the disrespect paid to her, by Printing the Cloaths, and other things were to be sent to her by the French King.[158] I told her the great fear of people was the Prince of Wales, she said there was none; That the Stocks fell, she said they would rise again. I told her not to be disquieted because most believ'd Her good design to the Kingdom, but the blame was laid upon the Ministry, as it ought, if they advis'd her, to any thing to her dishonour, or the disadvantage of the Kingdom.

30th. I read to the Queen the paper[159] which was spread up and down, To which she reply'd, There was nothing in it. I said their fear, was the Pretender. Reading the substance of my Lord Rivers's first Audience[160] to the Elector of Hanover as it was reported, viz, to assure him, that care should be taken to secure his Succession in England, and to have the 9th Electorate acknowledg'd, in the insuring Treaty with Spain. The Electors Answer. *And shall not I be Elector of Hanover, and shall not my Familly Succeed in England, unless the King of France pleases, let Spain be restored to the House of Austria, and respective Barriers be given to the Emperour, and Holland, and I shall Trust to Almighty God, the justice of my Cause, and the laws of Great Britain.* Telling her also what Lord Cowper said. The beginning of this Treaty, seems to be carry'd on, by a good correspondance with France; and with the dislike of the rest of the Confederacy. That if it terminate in the same manner, the Allies being disoblig'd, and France pleas'd, The Consequence is certain, that her Majesty's Reign, as well as any advantage France shall give us in the treaty, trust be held and continu'd to us at the Will of France, or while[l] France pleases, since none of the Allies can think themselves Concernd to support us.

December 4th. Discoursing with the Queen about the Bishop of Salisbury's Sermon, at Mercers Chappell,[161] saying there was as much danger of Popery now, as in the time of Popery, and that if the French King is Strengthned he will bring in the Pretender Even while the Queen is alive, and she will not be able to hinder it.

6th. Meeting my Lord Cowper, he said the Queen told him, there would be no Stop of endievour nor no cessation of arms, so that if it did not produce a peace, it might make the rest of the Allies bring in their Quotas.[162]

7th. Visiting the Queen, I told her, my Lord Cowper said, he saw the same goodness in her as before, and he hop'd that if Peace did not come, the Quotas of the Allies would be a good Effect of her Endeavour. That no body spoke well of Harley but Her Self.

8th. Vid: what Lord Harvey said.[163]

10th. I told the Queen that the first part of the Speech was objected against, as not being suitable to her Calm Temper, and that the French King had used the Expression to Cardinal Noailles in his letter. She said they were the words of the Common Prayer.[164]

Visiting Lord Cowper that day he gave this reason of Mr. Harleys failing the 2nd Day of Voting the Address with advice to the Queen, because says he, we see not as God, who sees all things at once, we fix on things singly,[m] so they that found themselves lose it by one fix'd their thoughts on making up that one,[165] sought

[l] or while] (*X*) when (*M*) [m] singly] (*X*)

Lord Carmarthen[166] and thought to have got Lord Hunsdon,[167] who wou'd not Unless they doubled his Pension,[168] so he came now. They did not consider the whole to Secure them again,[169] and the Vote was different, not whether to advise the Queen that it was not safe to yeild Spain to any branch of the House of Bourbon, but to Vote the approbation of drawing up what was advised. So when the Vote was carry'd by the Majority, it wou'd have lookd Ill not to approve the Comittee for doing that which they were directed[n] to do. He said that Part of the Speech, look'd like a Libeller in a Garret, with a Reflection on a General; and not like a Queen, who shoud not have thunder'd in that way. That word is Us'd against the French King, and not against those, that fight against him; That it looks Strange that the Ministry shoud desire time to Consider what they had Avis'd the Queen to. They ought to have Consider'd it well before they had dar'd to advise it.[170]

13th. In Converse with the Queen, I told her of the Reference to her Speech to the Allies, or the Duke of Marlborough, whereas in the Prayers it refferd to the French King. That it was mean for her to say so from the Throne, it was fitter in her chamber. That Mr. Harley while she was present spoke nothing, but once about the Order of the House, and then my Lord Sunderland told him he knew the contrary to be true,[o] to which he did not reply.[171] And that it was pittifull to desire time, to consider, when they shoud have consider'd before advising her Majesty.

14th. I told her that Lord Cowper press'd that care shoud be taken to have the Allies enlarge their Charge to the lessening of ours. Else he woud recede from the Vote.[172]

15th. This I told the Queen, and that it woud lessen our Charge two Millions, which woud be a good Effect of the Negotiations if Peace was not. My Lord Cowper being desirous of her having the Honour of making Peace, and of Her making Proposals. She said he made a peevish Speech yesterday, but did not remember the Parts of it.[173] She told me Lord Powlet[174] said there was no Credit in gaigning a Question when it was not debated to which my Lord Cowper answer'd that it was debated, only they who had nothing to say, Hitt on forms and words.[175] That it was Mr. Harleys

[n] directed] (*X*) desir'd (*M*)
[o] true] (*X*) false (*M*)

Misfortune that St. Johns high and Lord Keeper who took Fees of little Lords was with him,[176] that if the Duke of Newcastle had liv'd[177] or my Lord Cowper had joind, things had not come to this Conclusion. I said my Lord Cowper was against the Peace in his Opinion, and Acts according to it; which is better than One changing to, and fro; its that Temper which keeps up Divisions and makes Persecution, They say Your Majesty Equivocates by saying you'd endeavour to restore Spain, when its not thought of in the Preliminarys the Bill was brought in to make.[178]

I wish'd my Lord Cowper was in she said it was impossible. Visiting Lord Cowper and taking notice of the Reason of his going out, he said he saw it woud be a Tory Ministry, that woud carry it so high with Hereditary Right and Passive Obedience, that he could not join in it; tho' Mr. Harley said it would be a Whig Ministry, it woud be out of his Power to make it so.[179] That now he could not, because of the strengthning the hand of the French King and the Pretender. But the best Method would be to begin some days after the Congress upon the Old Preliminarys;[180] that it lessen'd the Queen, that Mr. St. John should let the Electors Memorial lie by, and yet be printed as soon as the Queen saw it.[181]

17th. Visiting the Queen, I told her that I understood my Lord Nottingham[182] had promis'd his Vote against the Peace; if they woud not Vote for the bill.[183] She said that will hurt no body as it is, but the Name of it frights people. I told her that people were so Alarm'd, that yesterday they preach'd Unitedly against Popery. To which she said They do such Things on Purpose to make confusion. I told her also I understood that the only way to hinder it from passing was by my Lord Bulingbrokes clogging it,[184] my Lord Nottingham having said he woud not Vote for it any other way than as it was drawn up.[185] The Queens answer shows how ignorant they kept her, particularly as to those who were Chiefly concernd in the bill.

20th. Visiting Her, She told me the bill woud hurt none but the Zealous Presbyterians. That she was going to the House upon Duke Hamiltons affair[186], saying 'twas pitty the Prerogative should be so Lessen'd.

27th. I express'd my self griev'd to see her so disturd [*sic*] between Partys abroad and Partys in her family. I do believe that the Visible Differences, made most thinking People commiserate Her Majestys

Circumstances in the Difficulty how to Act between; therefore beg'd she woud not be disquieted.

29th. I repeated my concern at the disquiet she had, and told her that two Suggestions might be of use to her. (1stly) that if the Ministry presum'd to disquiet her, by telling her, how they would leave Her, as was reported[187] she shou'd at least seem to accept of their offer, their Levées woud soon Link, and the respect they had upon the Account of Her Service woud soon diminish, that they woud be calld to an Account by the Whiggs whom she shoud be oblig'd to make succeed in their Places. (2ndly) to Prevent her being teas'd with family disquiets, to acquaint the Persons who did it, that nothing lessen'd love like the Objects of it giving disquiet. This was what lessend Her Affection for the Duchess of Marlborough, and would again do the same to those who gave her Uneasiness. But I must say Her Majesty was to me a Pattern of Patience, and her Bearing so much turn'd her into a Subject to be affraid, instead of a Queen to Cause Terrour in Others. This I can demonstrate by letting the whole world know, that she had deny'd Even Her own Inclinations, that she might not provoke those about her, and so by the Provocation be made uneasie in Her own Mind, which often forc'd her to have conversation with me Incognito both to keep Her Self Quiet, and me from being injur'd, which she often said to my self was Pitty, when I sought no by-End, but only aim'd at her Health and Quiet.

Is not what I have said demonstrated when I say, that if some Persons had been in waiting, however Her Majesty inclin'd to speak to me, yet either the Door must be left Open, or if that shut, I to stay no more than a Minute; whereas if others who had a Personal regard for me, had been then in waiting the door might be Shut, and I stay without her Concern. How often have Such Expressions grievd my mind as from a Queen, upon my attempting to kneel in reading any thing I had to say, No, somebody will come in; and upon Expectation of some Person appointed who might have made ill Use of my being with her, tho' I had Converse with none but her self and that without any By-end, yet she must be in danger of disquiet from it.

31st. Upon Her Majesty's asking, Did any body say anything of the twelve Lords,[188] I only answer'd that Day, that I heard it openly said, that it was done to turn out dutyfull Servants,[189] and that my Lord Oxford pack'd Jurys to carry Causes. That my Lord Hervey said it was unpresidented, that neither Edward the 2nd. nor Henry the 8th., That no Arbitrary or ruin'd Government ever did it; and that if Her Majesty's Father had done it he had sat upon the Throne.[190] Indeed said he, to do it when one comes to the Throne, to make them the better belov'd by their People, its well Enough; but to do it afterwards, and at such a Time, looks as if the Cause were weak. She desir'd me to obtain the thoughts and opinion of a Particular Person,[191] to which I reply'd that I would Certainly do it; but that it woud do Her greater service if she had that Persons Opinions Upon the first Motion of any thing to her, that so from Contrary reasoning, she might with the greater advantage Conclude what to do. And this would at least have two very good Effects as to Her Self: (1) it would hinder them from Acting by way of Imposition, and informing Her of Falshoods (2ndly) Her Judgement woud be strong, that they coud not so Easily resist it. To which she answered that tho' she could trust me, yet she was afraid to trust the Person I consulted, least they Vented it. I said I shoud be sure to let her know that Persons Opinion.

1712.

January 2nd. Having Obtain'd this Persons Opinion, I put it down in Paper and read it to Her Majesty. The step of Chusing 12 Lords, said he, is a legal Act of Her Majesty, but it is Us'd to an Extravagant Excess, and to a bad End; viz. the Modelling one of the Houses of Parliament; and that while Sitting which makes it still worse. This is Evident to every reasonable Person who considers the Circumstances of the Act. It follows upon two Divisions of the House, wherein the Credit of the Ministry was greatly concern'd and wherein they lost; so tis plain, it is not to reward Merit, (the End for which that Prerogative is trusted in the Crown) but to make Votes and Numbers. This is a Violation of the freedom of Parliaments; and such a thing as in all its Circumstances was never done before.

The Resolution was taken but on fryday. And they are to sitt on Wednesday. It's done to save a Ministry. To advise the Queen to a legal Act to a bad Purpose is Culpable.

I told her also that some talk'd so boldly, as if this was like to a Packing of Jurys to take away life, to all which Her Majesty answerd that King William made more;[192] to which I reply'd, that it was said, that that was not done at one time, and therefore it was plain that this[p] was not to reward Merit, but to make Votes. She said it was their own Fault, and told me the Duke of Marlborough was out; for he had not carry'd himself Well to her Majesty since he came home. That she did not mean to her Personally, but in her business.[193]

8th. Presented Her with the Advertisement about Prince Eugenes Mother.[194]

10th. I Presum'd to tell her; that if she had a liking to the Duchess of Sommerset it was Pity she did not Act her Own Will. For she needed an Agreable Friend to Open to, in Order to lessen the Ill Effects of Her Disquiets. And if she did not use her Own Power to keep in the Duchess of Sommerset for her Own quiet, it would give the Duchess of Marlborough a handle to say, that it was not her Fault that her Majesty parted with her, but her Majesty's Circumstances which occasion it. The Queen asking what I was talking before I came in, I told her it was about Mr. Beck,[195] whom Dr. Arburthnot[196] said he heard was a great Party Man; and was at pains to write over Affairs to Holland, which was odd, he being a Stranger and Unacquainted with the Laws of the Nation. But the Queen had a friendship for him, because he had done her some service, and had reccommended an Affair to Her out of Personal Respect to her.

23rd. In Converse with her Majesty, she express'd Her desire that the Duchess of Somerset Shou'd be kept in.[197]

24th. She Order'd me to go to My Lord Cowper to use all Interest with the Duke of Sommerset, that his Lady might continue Her Charge, she told me that the Arguments I shou'd Use, were her Health, which would be greatly Impar'd, if it happen'd that the Duke woud not let her Stay in. I told Her that yesterday upon discoursing it with my Lord Cowper, he told me, that he had prevaild with my Lord Duke at least as to[q] the removing of the Dutchess. But going this morning in Obedience to the Queens Commands, He told me the Duke of Sommerset was to be with him at Eleven, and he woud use his Endeavour.

Visiting my Lord at night, in order to acquaint Her Majesty next morning he told me that he had good hopes the Duke of

[p] this] (*X*) it (*M*) [q] as to] (*X*)

Somerset would be prevail'd upon, The Duke insisting upon his honour, and disreputation,[198] as if it was for money, and that upon my Lord Cowpers speaking to some Lords who were against her Stay, there was Suspition, that they would force the Queen to put her out again.

25th. Visiting the Queen I told her how ready my Lord Cowper was to Act, Especially upon Understanding the Queens Sincere Kindness to the Dutchess of Somerset, and that her going out would greatly disquiet her Majesty, and injure her Health. That he undertook to do all in his Power. That last night I Stay'd at his house till near Twelve when he came from the Parliament, and then he told me he had good hopes that the Duke would be prevail'd Upon. He insisted on his Honour as concernd in taking the Duchess away, least if he did not, people shoud think it was the gain of the Post for such[r] he had permitted her to Stay. He had Consulted several Lords who were against her Staying in, Saying that when her Majesty was gratified with the Duchess's Stay, then she woud turn her out. So that this was a lesson to Her Majesty to show Openly a Favour to those she thought merited it, whether the Ministry lik'd it, or not, for she saw that, that Suggestion Prevail'd that however people faithfully Serv'd Her, and however much Favour she show'd them; yet, if any Person next to Her, or that had any opportunity to Speak and Impress her, shoud say any thing against them, they would be turn'd out, and afterwards Disgrac'd. But when you fix your Favour right, and Maintain it, every Person must be fond of having it; and Faithfully Serve You in the Enjoyment of it. The Duchess of Somerset your Majesty has a respect for. She is of the first Quality and in that respect Suitable to You.[199] She seems to Converse with a Courteous Calmness which makes her the more Suitable to your Majesty's Temper.[200] But I hop'd she had an Openess to draw Your Majesty outward, and to Open to Her what are your Majestys Disquiets. Else your Majesty's Reserv'dness and Secrecy, might lose to you the greatest pleasure of Conversation. Her Majesty told me the Duchess was to have come yesterday at five if she had any good done. But she not comming the Queen wrote to Her, that by her not comming she suppos'd she had no good news,[201] and therefore desird her not to come till this day at five; that So, my

[r] for such] (*X*) for which (*S*)

Lord Cowper might have opportunity to influence the Duke of Somerset before the Duchess waited upon the Queen, desiring me to Visit Lord Cowper at night and hear what had Pass'd, and to come to her to morrow after the rest of the Phisitians were gone. Upon which I begg'd Her Majesty to be Easie; she answerd she would do all in her Power to be so.

The[n] Visiting according to the Queen's Commands Lord Cowper at night, His Lordship had had full time with the Duke of Somerset that Day; and told me that he found him comming and did not dout but he would come to a good Resolution. My Lord Cowper pressing first her Graces Stay, and at least a prolongation, especially if the Queen continu'd in kind condescension to desire it; for her Majestys perseverance therein, was a proof of Her real kindness and gave Hope that it woud continue; and so that objection of fearing the Duchess's being put out again by Persons Influence upon the Queen and that the Duke took Ill the harshness of some Expressions in the Letter, and in the way of putting him out. But my Lord Cowper told him, it was done on purpose to irritate him, and provoke him to take the Duchess away. That Lord Cowper design'd to take off the Lords who gave the Duke Ill impressions, that so, he might have their joint Opinion, with His, for her staying in. He telling me at the same time, that the Duchess's affection to the Queen was great; and made her free from all Resentment of putting out the Duke, and endeavour to convince him, that it was the necessity of the Queen's Affairs.

26th. Visiting the Queen, I read to her what had passd last night with Lord Cowper. Which (to show her great Caution) she made me burn before I went out of the room, for fear of accidents. Her Majesty told me the Duchess had been with her yesterday at five according to her appointment, and told her the Duke was more likely to Yeild. But because the Queen imagin'd that Lord Cowper was likely to speak to the Duke at the House, and that the House sitting late,[202] the Duke would not be able to see the Duchess before she waited on her at five. Therefore the Queen had put it of till the 26th. at five, If there was any good to be done, or Else about nine with a final Resolution. And desird me to get Lord Cowper to use his Endeavour to day. The Queen also said that What she wrote to the Duke woud not seem harsh, if he showd it to any body. Viz. that nothing but himself could have made him be out.

Then Visiting Lord Cowper, according to the Queen's command; he told me that at Noon he heard the Duke's resolution was to let the Duchess stay in. The Duke saying to Lord Cowper that His Lordship woud take this as an Eminent Instance of the Dependance he had upon his Judgement, it being by his sole Perswasion, and he hop'd that if he heard him blam'd he would Vindicate him. My Lord telling me at the same time, that it was Fitt, the Queen shoud be prepard, for their Endeavours against the Duchess, in which they had already begun, by the Windsor Prophecy:[203] Saying she was an Assassin in her Youth, and would Poison the Queen in her more grown Years.[204] And the Duke knew it to be a design to Lessen her, and to make her fall a sacrifice to Mrs. Massam; because Swift was notoriously Employ'd by the Ministry.[205]

27th. Being Sunday I did not Visit the Queen But on

28th. Monday going into the Queen after the Duchess of Somerset came out from Her, I never saw the Queen Look with a more pleasant and Healthfull Countenance, saying that Now, it was done. After Expressing my Joy that the Affair was fix'd, I told her Majesty what had pass'd between the Duke of Somerset and my Lord Cowper; and what had pass'd between my Lord Cowper and me, on Saturday. And Also of their Fear, least the Queen should be turn'd from Her, because this day they had been endeavouring to bespatter Her by the Windsor Prophecy, and so might go on to do so still. She said, that woud have no Influence on her, to turn Her respect from the Duchess. I told her that upon my saying the Same, I was answer'd, that it had happen'd So, between Her Majesty, and others, to which she said, That that was owing to the Duchess of Marlborough's own Temper and Cariage, and she was sure, she would never meet with any such thing from the Duchess of Somerset.

29th. I show'd her Majesty the Windsor Prophecy, which she declin'd to see. A reproof to Others, that delight to Read, and Hear Reproaches, and charg'd me not to mention to any one, that I had mention'd it. I begging Also, that I might not be known in any faithfull Service of mine. That being all I aim'd at, the maintaining her health and quiet of mind; and the knowing what Others said in Order to direct her Judgement. I had no Vanity to be spoke of as having the Honour of Serving Her Majesty, for the Malice it would draw upon me would Lessen the Pleasure of It.

30th. Between the 30th. January and the 14th February a Feavour, but

February 15th. Visiting the Queen the 15th. she discours'd of Dr. Swifts Character. He was good for some things she said But had not dispos'd of that Benefice to him, nor woud not.[206]

19th. In Converse with Her Majesty. I gave her my own Private Opinion against that part of the Bill, for Toleration in Scotland;[207] by which all Power was taken away from the Magistrates to exercise their Authority against Immorality. Punishing Imorality was the Cause of God Almighty; and I thought the restraining that, could not be very pleasing to a Pious Queen if it was rightly imparted to Her. She said those things bore different Interpretation.

20th. Visiting the Queen. Pleased to see that Devoutness she Exercis'd in Her Closet. From this to April the 5th. confin'd to bed; and was not able to attend Her Majesty till May.

May 5th. Visiting the Queen She discours'd with me concerning the Reformation of Manners,[208] and my Spirit being then more than ordinary Serious, just as it were risen from the dead, after being given over by all, I told Her, what a Mercy it was She had so many Instruments of doing good in the Nation, who not only appointed Times of United Prayer for their own success, but Hers also; and were ready to do it also for Her Life and Health, when Sick.

19th. Her Majesty being desirous I shoud not wait upon Her too often till I had recover'd my Strength I had not now such frequent returns of Discourse. But this day gave Her my Lord Cowpers compliments, for not waiting on her before He went out of town; as also told her, of the great Advantage of Friendship in point of Health and quiet of Mind, asking if Her Majesty did not think Her Satisfaction in the Duchess of Somerset, did not contribute to Her Health. She said Yes, I mentioning some secret disquiets I had, which had a contrary Effect upon me, and keeped me back from recovring Strength.[209]

June 7th. In Converse with Her, She said She hop'd the Peace would be a good Peace, and sent for every body to town, naming my Lord Harvey.[210] Upon which I said, I hop'd she would be honour'd to make a good Peace in Reward to Her Pious Life.

12th. In Converse with the Queen, she said Lord Cowpers reasons, in converse with Her were so weak that a man of his sence could not believe them.[211] That he spoke in the House as any.[212] That

Dunkirk was matter of fact,[213] as well as the Towns which were to be given at the last Treaty.[214]

July 14th. I told Her that I believ'd this of Dunkirk would quiet a great many Peoples Minds, who were Uneasie before, but that the Most Pious, who were not in Party, nor Faction, were concern'd least there was a design to bring in the Pretender. Their Arguments for this were, the Treatment given to the Elector of Hanover: to which she said His Treatment to me, had not been Civil, if I had done or Treated King William my Predecessour so, it would have been thought so. Another Argument is because theres a report, that he has an English Divine for His Chaplain; and His Servants Protestants and Himself to be a pretended Protestant. She said there was no Protestant Chaplain with him, and He himself was to be sent away.[215] Then I told Her they said that Tho' his coming in might not be directly with Her consent, Yet they might bring Her to do Such Things, as would Neccessarily force Her to yeild to it. To which she said, Can any think me so blind as not to see through these Things. I told Her this Story spread was the Chief thing to be suppress'd, she said that was now a doing. I said I hoped the same Providence which had made Her so Successfull in Warr, would Also make Her Successful in Framing a Peace.

21st. See the Care she took to give Trouble to Dr. Keith's[216] Friend that notwithstanding her Affairs, she shoud remember to send to my lodgings that she was gone to Town, That so, the Person might not lose her Favour in comming to be touch'd.

29th. Then going to the Queen at Windsor, I told Her that I had made Impression Upon Some, by that Expression of Hers to abate their Anger, That if She had done that to King William which the Elector did to Her, she would have been blam'd, she said Time would bring them to Reason.

September 9th. Visiting the Queen at Windsor She told me there was nothing in it, as to the Pretender, and desir'd that none might impose upon me such Impressions. She might Trust Providence to Preserve Her life from Evil Hands, and what I had said, she took in the right Sence I telling Her that the Evening Post last Saturday said that the Pretender call'd himself Duke of Glocester. She ask'd if it was in the Post boy.[217] I told Her my concern was least mentioning the Succession of the Pretender After Her, they would not wait, but Poison Her, she knowing they would Judge the Fact Meritorious, and deserving Heaven. She discour'd also the Story of Mr. St. Johns being at the Play with the Pretender;[218] she said He ought to have gone Out Immediatly,[219] and Upon my saying it was talk'd that Dr. Swift was to be Dean of Wells,[220] she said it was false, and desir'd that nothing they said might Impress me.

17th. I came to Windsor and the Queen Ill, so there was no Opportunity of Converse.

27th. Visiting the Queen at Windsor I told Her how concern'd People were about the Pretender, as also Her Sickness.

October 8th. Visiting Lord Cowper he said things were much worse than when he left them. They had made the Queen contradict Her self in all Her Speeches, Treacherous to Her Confederates, and made France Triumphant over the Allies,[221] and when he had dealt with them, he would deal with us and fix the Pretender on the Throne. They endeavourd to make Her believe he had a right. If he has he should have immediate actual Possession. Will she who holds the Crown to support the Protestant Interest, give it up to a Popish Prince, when she can hold it no longer, by reason of Death. They may make believe that they'll stay till Her Death, but the Roman Catholicks never miss'd their Opportunity, and Will either give her foul Play, or bring him in, whether she will or not. And that If by putting all his Friends in Posts, Modelling a Parliament and Army for it,[222] how then can she hinder it, she can only say she expected no such Treatment. They let in King Charles to every Part of the Plot but what related to his Own life.[223] What shame it is that in all the Addresses from the Countrey they Extol this Ministry for Extending trade to Parts formerly unknown to the English Nation[224]. And what is all this come to, to blind the world with a Shadow, buying up Goods as if they were a going to the South-Sea, and forc'd now to sell them for 20 per Cent loss.[225] How dos the Cessation of Arms promote Trade, when the trading Merchants to Portugal, must ly still, unless they venture being taken by the French.[226] England is oblig'd not to send Convoys thither with them, nor to trade with their Enemys, but the Kingdom is so secure and so blind, that they believe any thing. If when the Parliament meets they say it is no Seperate Peace, thats like Killigrew who laid a Wager with King Charles, that he would not wear a Vest, a twelvemonth and so[s] he wore a Short coat, before the Year was out, and Killigrew desir'd to have his Wager. But says the King it is a Vest.[227] Ah says he I will never lay a Wager with a King, again. So He'll say its no Separate Peace. The Independent Enthusiasticks took away King Charles life[228] Openly but the French and Papists do all by Stabbing. Honour is lost to make the King of France Triumphant, and made so great Successes against him, and when he was truckling to the Confederates to break the Confederacy, and to let in Bitterness amongst them against each other, to withdraw all Troops and Ships and to leave them to the Fury of the Enemy, and what Unfaithfulness to Solemn Alliances, after the Queen's Saying she would take care of the Confederates. And of the Flying-post talking that the Pretender was call'd the Duke of Gloscester.[229] How can that be cur'd but by entering into the warming Pan again.

11th. Visiting at Windsor I told the Queen that I had seen my Lord Cowper, who was concern'd to hear that she had been ill[230] and told me that Things look'd as tho' the Pretender was design'd, and all in Places, who are for him. Oh fye says she, there is no such thing. What, do they think I'm a Child, and to be imposed upon, and that I have only Integrity? I said to Her, I was sure Her Majesty was not in the Pretenders Affair, and that I hop'd she would live long to Prevent it. I challeng'd my Lord for not waiting oftner on Your Majesty to Show his Affection and his being of no Party. To which she said he was as much so as any man. If he Visited Your Majesty often they would say he was a going of, giving her an instance of their report of Mr. Steele[231] as such, upon his going two or three times to my Lord Oxford. I have endeavour'd to impress Mr. Steele with an Assurance of Your Majestys not being in the Pretenders Interest. He said if he thought that, he woud goe home and sleep sounder than he had done for many nights. I ask'd Her if I said any thing I ought not. She said No, but the less I talkd with them, the better.

November 8th. The Queen mention'd the Box which was sent to my Lord Oxford, with a Pistol in it.[232] And of my Lord Marlboroughs going abroad. She said it was prudent in him.[233]

22nd. At Windsor, I told the Queen that previous to every Preferment in the Degrees of Her Establishment, I had a fitt of sickness always to Prepare me for it. Telling Her also my belief, that the Pretender

[s] twelvemonth and so he] (*M*) twelvemonth, he (*X*)

was not the real son of King James with my Arguments against it, that there was no weight to be laid upon the Particular Depositions of the Birth but upon Mrs. Wilkes's the Midwife,[234] whose hand was to bring the Child out of the body. Her deposition to me is of no weight because she is a Roman Catholick; her Principles telling her how meritorious such an Act would be in another World; as well as her Interest Speaking How gainful it would be. Besides she has never been heard of since by any of her friends, Again, I have been Witness to the same imposition amongst Persons of a farr, less Degree, and to Answer a farr less design. All which, fix my Opinion at least, as to the Probability of the thing. Her Majesty received this with Chearfulness, and by asking me several questions about the Thing.

December 10th. Discours'd only of the Melancholiness of my Own Affair, and endeavour'd to take her advice of Privacy in the matter. But it was not to be done.[235]

13th. The Queen order'd me to tell my Lord Cowper how perfectly Well the Duchess of Somerset was with the Queen because it had been said, that after she was in they would endeavour to give bad Impression of Her. She told me also that Mackartney[236] was seen crossing to Putney 2 days ago.

18th. She told me the Duchess of Somerset was gone to Petworth with some concern, upon which I said I hop'd upon no discontents. To which she said not at all. The Queen having given me leave to inquire at any time of such a thing, that I might assure my Lord Cowper of the same who was at first so afraid of it.

19th. I only thank'd Her Majesty for giving me leave to mention any little concern of mine, which gave me trouble, and doing me the Honour to interest her self therein by advice, which I had found Successful. To which She Answerd, That it would make Her appear very Unkind after my showing so much Sincere Concern for her health and Quiet not to do it. This was from her self, and without the knowledge of Others, and every thing that came to me from her self was of the same sort So that I cannot but say that the Queen in her self had all the goodness of temper of Courtesy and breeding, of Compassion, and Inclination to serve the World, and what had another Appearance was from outward Influence, and none of the Queen not being Intimate with Such. I am not capable to accuse Particular Persons, but having spoke to, and known so much of the Queen, as to what sprung from her Self, I shoud be false in the highest degree, and Ungrateful to the Countenance she gave me, not to maintain to my last breath this Character of Her, to the honour of Her Memory.

22nd. Visiting the Queen it being munday, I told her I thought She look'd on Saturday as if something had troubled Her. I wish'd that the Duchess of Somerset had not gone. And here I cannot but take Notice, how every disquiet dwelt upon Her Self within and how unwilling she was to own it unless drawn by some Conversation which forc'd Her to it. This was what I was afraid of, as the only thing wanting in the Duchess of Somerset to make her a Suitable Perfect Companion to the Queen, a Temper free from meddling and prying into other peoples affairs tho' nearly related to her, and tho' this be Wisdom in its Self, and follow'd with the happy Effect of much Quiet of Mind, Yet with Respect to the Queen the Duchess being suitable in Quality, in Affection to Her Majesty and in this very sort of reservedness, it had been still happier for the Queen that her Grace had been more open, and presuming to ask, especially since her Asking would have been without any By-End, and only given relief to Her Majestys mind when she had so much uneasiness elsewhere from Other Hands. Theres none acquainted with Unbyass'd Affectionate friendship, but also know that the very presence of a Friend is a new Strength given to a Mind, tho' their conversation happen to be upon the most common Things: which made me often suggest to the Dutchess, that she should be as much with the Queen as possibly her circumstances would permit. This I did with the Queens allowance, Tho' sometimes to Her Graces wondering, she not knowing my unbiass'd concern for the Queen at that time. None acquainted with this sort of Friendship, but if standing by Her Majestys bed side in her last Sickness, and observ'd the Soft Courteous way of the Duchess's speaking to the Queen and Her Majestys look and Motion of Her face in receiving it, tho' so Ill, and without sometimes answering a word, but must have seen a solid inward Satisfaction in the Duchess's Presence with Her.[237] It is not much talking, professing, and Promising, that are the Effects of such a liking, an Inward Suitableness of Temper, and a fix'd, Solid, calm, Friendship the Effect of it appears in a silent Gesture, as much as the other, in all its outward Motions Spending its Self, into Decay thereby, while the other is Supported by a Meer Union of the Soul and an Inward Delight from thence.

I told Her Majesty she was teaz'd to preffer Dr. Swift, and said that in conversation, I did not contradict it, because such a report look'd well on her Side, and it made it look the better that their Teazing did not make her yeild. Obtaining an Appointment for my Lord Cowper to wait upon her at five, and telling Her what a Personal regard he had always for Her, and how pleas'd he was to Serve her Personaly, but that he could not help his being in his Opinion against their Measures for if he was to be torn asunder for it he must say that they had betrayd Europe. To which she said That when one was in a Party, it was the Influence of That, that guided their Discourse and Opinion, and till he show'd himself by his Actions not to be in a Party, She could not trust his Opinion.

24th. Her Majesty desir'd me to tell Lord Cowper, not to say She sent for him, To which I said, that he had Truth enough of his Side to say that he came to know of Her Health.

27th. She complain'd that my Lord Cowper stay'd so little a while, An Argument of Her liking his conversation. I excus'd it from my Lords apprehending Her in pain at the time he was with Her. She said She saw he was in the Party, by his Vindication of Mackartney; and telling Her how impossible it was for[t] Captain Hamilton,[238] not to fall upon Mackartney, or to desire him to be taken Up. My Lord also saying He hop'd the Ministry would make use of this, to save persons from Dueling, by making it a law, that those who contributed shou'd have no Grace from the Crown and those that fought, shoud never be capable of Any Place.[239] I begg'd leave to write to the Duchess of Somerset of Her Majestys having the Gout[240] since she went, which she forbid by saying she had wrote on tuesday, and a Servant wrote every day to Her.

30th. Complimenting Her Upon the Dutch coming into the Peace,[241] I wish'd Smiling Providences might accompany so Pious a Life as Hers. For if otherways I was satisfy'd it was from the failure of others about Her and not from Her Self, to which she said she hop'd in Time that satisfaction woud be brought about to every body.

31st. Visiting the Queen I took notice to Her Majesty that I imagin'd Her fitt was a beginning on Saturday, when she seemd to be disquieted.

[t] impossible . . . for] (*X*) unanswerable . . . in (*M*)

I did not know but disquiet might forward it, and told Her that If I had met Mrs. Massam, or my Lord Oxford that Day, I could not have help'd talking to them, to keep of Business, and Especially Disquieting Business; She answer'd Softly, that I need not do that. To which I replyd that she kept all within, whereas nothing was so injurious as Disquiet lodg'd within ones self. I also said that the Duchess of Somersets calmness, made Her a most suitable companion to Her Majesty. To which She said, So She is.

Telling Her, how often I mention'd to Mrs. Danvers,[242] that if I ever askd any thing from the Queen it should be with the Condition, if she could grant it without uneasiness to Her self. But I was afraid she might be forc'd to do things Uneasie to Her Self to gratify the Inward Presentiments of others, and their cravings after gains, and honour, whether it was follow'd with Disquiet to Her or not. At the same time I presum'd to say that if the Duchess of Marlborough had been of the Temper of the Duchess of Somerset, She had never gone Out. No, says She.

1713.

January 1st. Discourse of Lady Ashburnham[243] taking Medecines from Mrs. Cotton,[244] when with Child, and that that was her disease etc., was only a Story of Hers.

2nd. Discourse of Mr. Becks[245] coresponding with the Secretary of Hanover[246] if it would give Her any Pleasure or do Her any Service, She desir'd that nothing might be ask'd of him to do, but if he of himself mov'd it, it would do well enough. I told Her that they were impress'd, Yea the Elector himself that she would be prevail'd upon to give Up the Crown—That came only from Holland, after its being writt to them from hence. There were many things said of the Elector, that were not true. You may Answer Every body, that that cannot be, besides that she is not press'd to any such thing.

8th. Telling Her how right Her judgement was as to Dr. Chamberlain,[247] because I had look'd over the Bills, and there was none writt by him for my Lady.

12th. Discoursing my own Experience of the good Effect of Converse with a Friend in a difficulty of mine, that I could not forbear renewing quiet of Mind, as well as Motion for Her Health, and that as one way to obtain it renewing to Her the Success she had with this when Lord Godolphin took care to keep of Usual

Occasions of Disquiet from Her, and when the Duchess of Somerset attended her Closely at Windsor, presuming to press Her Majesty not only to be pleas'd with Such Occasions, but to endeavour to have them. There was often a Friendship between Persons without suitableness, but in Her friendship with the Duchess, there was a suitableness of Quality, of Temper calm, and of breeding and Natural Affection, which makes the Friendship much more comfortable without interruption and lasting, an unsuitableness in any one thing, often breaking forth, Especially if in opinion, unless the Person resolve never to speak of that thing wherein there is an Unsuitableness, as was the Duchess's Prudence, besides she never press'd the Queen Hard, nothing makes the Queen more Uneasie than that.

17th. Coming into the Queen after the Duchess came out, was pleas'd, and discours'd of Her with the same pleasure.

19th. Discours'd about the Verses on Duke D'Aumont.[248] Her Majesty saying that He sold no Wine, she also shewing pleasure in Discoursing of the Duchess of Somerset, and saying she was 2 years younger than the Queen etc. which is one of the proofs of sincere affection a delight to talk of them when out of the Presence.

20th. The Queen said that she had seen the Paper in which the Duchess was reflected,[249] and that now there was a great many Scurilous papers that reflected Upon Her, such as the Flying-Post.[250] I told her my Lord Cowper burnt it after he read it, and that he said it was not to be allow'd, and that he had a Personal Affection to Her, to which She reply'd that Well then, Show it, but in the Parliament he is as Hot as any. Telling Her also that two things were neccessary qualifications in all about the Queen, Personal Affection, and soft smooth Treatment.

21st. Discoursing of the flying Post I told the Queen the only way to suppress the flying post would be by Suppressing the Examiner; she said he had been rebuk'd, but they will be taken notice of, and then told her that in Print was mention'd a Lord that had no Issue, and was Gouty, to Settle his Estate upon a Popish Heir, I did believe that Proceeded from the discourse of Searching for King Henry 8ths. Will; as a Precedent for Her Majesty to do it, and so if that power be given you, you may turn it to the Settling as they say you did of the late Ministry tho' You approv'd of them, alterd and turn'd them out. I told Her Lord Hervey said that of the 13 millions is [?][u] Lord Nottingham has 6, she said he had many thing[s] to say of Her besides That.[251]

22nd. Showing the Queen the Paper resembling Her to King Asa, and the Gouty foot.[252] Asking Her also if presents came from France to Her. Discoursing the thirteen Millions rais'd Tho' in Time of Peace, of which no Account can be given, telling Her that all this Proceeds from their Jealousy of the Pretender. Then Discoursd the Bishop of Salsiburys book that was come out, wherein he says then when he Ordain'd some Clergymen, he finds them such as shoud go back to Study, in order to be Capable to receive the Lords Supper.[253] To which she replyd, He knows all Things, and says more than any body, and that last Summer he said the Pretender would be Here before six weeks.

26th. Telling Her, how affectionately Lord Cowper spoke against the book, when I showd him about King Asa, he saying they would impress her as if it was from the Whigs.

February 2nd. Discoursing the Queen, I told her that the Flying post had mentiond nothing since and that Upon my asking a fitt Time for Lord Cowper waiting upon her, she seemd to decline it, not so much from disregard to him, as for fear of giving Occasion of Suspicion to those about Her.

11th. She discoursd of Dr. Shadwell,[254] writing to the Duke and Duchess of Shrewsbury how Ill she was desiring me to say to any, about her going to the house that she hopd to go in a Forthnight, to which I said, I hoped Sooner.

12th. She discours'd concerning what is in the Post-boy about Colonel Hamilton.[255] She wonder'd that it had not been done before, he having sworn it, soon after the Duke was killd. As also that if Lord Cowper ask'd to see Her of himself, I shoud tell him to call at any time, to ask how She did, but not to see Her, and not to do that till the week after the next, when the Duchess of Somerset would be out of Waiting, Least they shoud think there was Something between the Duchess of Somerset and him. To which I Replyd, that it was Pity she shoud not take so much Power as to see whom she pleas'd. But I saw her Natural Temper was calm, and since she was so unwilling to give any Uneasiness to Others Inferior to Her Self, it was Pity that all Inferiour to Her, and Under the Influence of Her Kindness shoud not keep her Easy.

[u] [?] *ms. illegible*. 'I have left out a word I could make nothing of' (*S*)

I wonder that Under the load of so much business, she could remember to Regulate, every such little Circumstance.

16th. Discoursing the Queen I told Her that Auditor Harley desir'd me to tell Her how much it was upon his Heart to have the Galley Slaves releas'd;[256] I shoud have done it sooner, but I was afraid he did it to try whether ever I spoke to Her Majesty. Fy No says She. Then I answerd that this was a Commendable Inclination in the Auditor, to which She said he was a very good man. I told Her also that I vented in all Companys that She was not in the Interest of the Pretender, and ask'd if I did well. To which She said Yes, you may so with the greatest truth, and seem'd exceedingly pleas'd when I told Her that Sir Richard Vivian[257] told me that he knew England so Well, especially the West of England, that they would turn against my Lord Treasurer as one man if there was any thing talk'd of the Pretender.

17th. In discourse with the Queen was mentiond Polignacs[258] having the Cardinals Cap by the Nomination of the Pretender. She answerd, Poor Creature, he has Influence to do Nothing.

25th. Mention'd Auditor Harleys letter, sent to my Lady Massam, about the release of the Galley Slaves.

March 2nd. Discoursd with me, Her Unwillingness to Save Mr. Noll,[259] because it was so barbarous a thing.

3rd. Went to the House.

6th. Discoursing the Queen I said that I hop'd after the Peace, *if it was a good One*, my Lord Cowper would be of no Party. She smiling said, That time would discover that. I said that Lord Oxford was a Secret man, and peoples not knowing the Springs of Actions and their Ends, made them talk differently, but I hoped all would be well at last, this she did not receive with her usual Satisfaction.

9th. I told Her persons were inquisitive at this time How her Spirits did, which made me afraid of Her having disquiets.

10th. Her Majesty said that it fell out well enough that my Lord Keeper was Sick, and also my Lord Trevor,[260] who she designd shoud Act in his room. I told Her that of all things She ought, especially to Guard against disquiet. I was sure she might do so if she pleas'd, for when she frown'd upon any one Person, every body Else did the Same. Instancing the Declention of my Lord Godolphins Attendance, when out of Her Employment. It was common in a little familly, when any one Child or servant was more regarded than the rest, each Envy'd, spoke and acted against that Person, who had the Favour, and to be Sure whoever has your Majestys Favour, they are Unwilling to lose it, and if Your Majesty tell them, that if you was disquieted by them it would be so, You woud have less of it. However it is ungenerous in any to Grudge others Your Majestys Favour, when they have a sufficiency of it to themselves. This comes of narrowness of Spirit, and largeness of Corrupt Appetites.

12th. I told Her it was reported that the Duke of Kent[261] and my Lord Dorset[262] had been with Her by Her Command, in Order to assure them there was nothing in the Pretender, but that She spoke so low about the Pretender that they could not tell what to make of it. To which she said that the Duke of Kent came of himself, and did they expect I shoud speak in a Passion.

13th. Upon asking a Convenient Time for my Lord Cowper, she told me that company came so much to Her, and she had so much to do, that she could not appoint a Time.

14th. Discoursing Her about an affair of my Own, I told Her that Mrs. Harley[263] ask'd me if the Queen knew it; I ask'd her, whether I shoud own it or be Silent. She commanded the latter, As an argument of her Secrecy in any Access she admitted me to.

17th. Visiting the Queen I told Her Lord Hervy ask'd me if a Person had not reason to be jealous of his wife if She was always endeavouring to prove Her own Chastity, asking me if it look'd Chaste in the Queen from the Pretender, to send for these Noblemen to Vindicate her self from being for the Pretender. I told Her that I replyd to this, that undoubtedly She had friends about Her, who, told her that it was reported that She was for the Pretender, and therefore it was neccessary to Vindicate her Self to Noblemen, that were against him, to remove their Ill impressions against Her, asking if I did aright, to which She said Very Right.

April 4th. Discoursing the affair of the Peace, I said I hop'd Her own Piety, and her Designs of Integrity for the good of Her People, woud be means of Producing good to the Nation, Unless the Nations Guilt, and the Disingenuity of the Ministry shoud Provoke God to permit it to be otherwise.

6th. I told Her that Stocks rose in the morning, and fell in the Afternoon by the Jews selling out.[264] Which made People Suspicious of their knowing something that might occasion it. That I found in all my Conversation, that if Her Majesty would give some Satisfaction to the people of Her not being for the Pretender, all would be easy. The Examiner seem'd to write in Order to take away such suspitions.[265] That I was told of a Report that Her Majesty woud mention somewhat in the House, of a friendship between Her and the Elector of Hanover but said at the same time it would be contradicted by the Elector. How can they say that, said She, when there is a good Understanding between the Elector and me. I told Her people were Shy of Speaking 'till Her Speech from the Throne,[266] but they still surmis'd there was something between the Treasurer and the French King which she did not know of. Who can help their Jealousies said She. I told Her that friends Vindicated Her, because her compliance was suitable to their Representations, and if any thing was acted wrong it was owing to them more than to Her. After Her Speech I said they would Open.

10th. I told Her that People were extreamly well pleas'd with that part of Her Speech, about the Protestant Succession, as also that part of it about rewarding Officers.[267] This woud beget Affection to Your Majesty. They debated the Address because they thought it woud be a Sanction to the Peace. Their Debate says she was very silly, when it was only to thank me.[268] I hear, said she, that Lord Cowper spoke against it. I said I shall hear his reasons, and make report to Your Majesty to Morrow.

Visiting Lord Cowper, he told me he only Spoke to one line, to Congratulate Her on Successful Endeavours to bring about a *General* Peace, which said He was a falshood.

11th. Upon giving Lord Cowper's Reason, she said, That was Only an Excuse, for it was a General Peace, the Emperour woud Certainly come in;[269] and said Lord Cowper shoud show his Affection to Her, in Actions as well as words.

12th. Discoursing their Desires to have the Treaty laid before them, she said She would only lay her Own, the others would be translated, and that would a little Stop their Surmises. I told Her that the way to remove the Notion of Whig and Tory, would be by having some Whigs as well as Tories in the Government, such as Lord Cowper. She said He's as hard as Steel, and you'll see, He will speak against my Affairs.

18th. Mentioning a Story of the Duchess of Somerset's going between the Queen and the Duchess of Newcastle,[270] in Order to get a Match between the Duke of Newcastles Daughter[271] and the Duke of Somersets Son.[272]

25th. She discours'd of Dr. Swifts being a Dean in Ireland, saying that all the Deanerys in Ireland were of the Lord Lieutenants gift, but the Bishopricks of Hers.[273] I told Her most knew that she was pressd to prefer him, and it was Honourable to Her as a Pious Queen, to refuse it. She said the Remonstrance of the Pretender[274] was forged in Holland and sent over here a Year ago, but was not given to the Plenipotentiarys but I told Her Lord Cowper said it was Genuine, and given to the Plenipotentiarys under a Cover.

29th. I beg'd Her care of Her Health; for if she happend to dye it was very probable that the Nation would be in blood; and to preserve Her Health there was nothing like quiet of Mind. Nothing could disquiet Her but two Things, either the Government which is left to the Ministry, or the Family; each of which she could frown down when she pleas'd.

30th. There being a Report that the Exchange of Ratifications was Stopp'd, I repeated my intreaty that she shoud not be disquieted, to which she reply'd, She had no Occasion to be disquieted upon that Account, because the Ratifications were exchang'd and woud be over in a Post.

May 1st. I told Her how few knew that Swift was prefferd by the Duke of Ormond,[275] and not by Her, but that I had remov'd the Mistake where I went, by what she told me Her self.

5th. I told the Queen that now Peace being concluded, Lord Oxfords next work, was to reconcile all Partys for Her quiet, with which She was well pleas'd, and told me the Emperours, always Stood out from coming in to a Peace.

6th. She asking me, what the City said, I told Her Stocks did not rise, because the Article of Commerce was not laid before the House,[276] and because it was not believed, that the Emperor would come in. She said the Emperour did not come in last time.

7th. She was extreamly well pleasd to hear what was told me, that the Treaty of Succession was, as it was, open'd by Mr. Moore,[277] and if upon Opening the Article of Commerce, it was, as it was said, we might hope well from it. Nothing pleas'd the Queen like telling her of the Satisfaction of the people; and that She did not Satisfy them was owing to telling Her, that they were Satisfied when they were not, for a few days before Her last Sickness, Her Conviction of the Disatisfaction of the People, out of a fear, of Her being in the Interest of the Pretender, bore harder upon Her, than all the Differences among her Ministers, as is commonly reported, which will appear from what follows.

8th. I told Her how lucky it was that she told me the Deaneries in Ireland were not in her Gift, for Neither Lord Kingston,[278] nor Lord Harvey knew it till I acquainted them. People Grumbled that the Articles were not Laid before the House; She said it took time to write over the Copies, and hoped by that time, and the Parliament reading them over, the Emperour would be come in, and so All would be at an End. I said Pious People, such as the Bishop of Norwich[279] were afraid of the French Kings Strength, to which She said, he was a very good Man, but guided by Lord Sunderland.

14th. I told Her Sir Richard Vivian said the Treaty of Commerce was Mysterious, and the Fish not going to France,[280] might ruine part of the Countrey.

19th. I told the Queen it was said, the goodness of the Peace woud be known by its fruits, by the Success of the Commissioners of Britain and France meeting here; that if Upright Designs had been pursu'd they might have been in the bowels of France; and then a good Peace might have happen'd.

June 1st. In her Uneasiness about the Scots proposing the Dissolution of the Union,[281] She told me my Lord Seafield,[282] was fitter than any one, to Open the thing in Parliament.

4th. Meeting Lord Marr[283] at the back Stairs, I desir'd him not to teaze the Queen, now the Gout was upon her, for what teaz'd the Queen weakn'd Her Spirits, whereas by the Strength of them Illness was to be thrown Outwards.

5th. Telling Her of my Converse with Lord Marr. She was pleas'd, but desir'd me to Speak no more to any of them.

6th. Visiting Her She told me there would be difficulty on Monday.[284]

8th. She told me that, what was done, was done, to hinder Business, and from Personal Disrespect to Her, to which I said, I hop'd it was rather to my Lord Oxford, but begg'd she woud not be disquieted Since the Event Happend on Her Side.

11th. The Queen said they were hot, but the Bill would be carry'd.

Visiting Lord Cowper that night, he said the Queen should be

Neuter, leaving the Matter to be battled, and debated in Parliament, without concern, and let right take Place, Else she makes her self Queen of a Party, and Her Ministers who shoud free Her, lay all the Weight Upon Her.

15th. Convers'd how injurious Disquiet was.

16th. She said there was some Comotion in Scotland, that Sir David Dalrymple[285] had come up Post for something, she suppos'd they had write for him. I said I shoud see him, and know why he came up, she said she suppos'd they would keep that close. Then meeting the Duchess of Somerset, I beg'd she would be with the Queen as much as she could, to which she said, to be sure she would if she thought it any wise for the Queens Advantage.

19th. She heard Sir David Dalrymple had spoke in the House.[286]

After this I was taken Ill, in which Illness I sent a letter to Introduce Mr. Ceasar[287] to the Queen and then making him set down in writing Arguments for the Queens Health.

July 6th. Visiting the Queen after my Recovry. I thank'd Her Majesty for giving the King of Prussia's Chaplain[288] so kind an access, for He saw her well, and would report it abroad, and he had from me some Arguments of her long life. I hop'd she had not been disquieted since my Illness. That I hopd she was sensible that endeavours were against Lord Oxford, and not against Her, and wish'd He was made sensible of two things, and that the Cry of these two things might Impress him. 1st. of promising, and not performing. 2ndly the Cry of the Poor for what is owing them. She said there had been such Vast occasions for money lately that he could not, but now this would pay the arrears, for there was no Debt since He came. To which I said it was mostly since he came, and it was pitty Lord Godolphins Memory should Suffer, and his Reputation to Stand on others Disreputation; for when he was put out[v] there was but one half year owing me, but now theres near three Years owing. So that it plainly appears Her Majestys forced, by Indisposition and returns of disquiet to trust others. She was kept not only from Persons of a Contrary Opinion, but from the Knowledge of things, and therefore her Ignorance, and progress suitable to that, is imputable to Others and not to Her. I advis'd Her not to go to Pauls, least she suffer'd in Her Health, but rather to St. James's,[289] and that would satisfy the People, and not injure Her.

[v] was put out] *Marginal note* (*M*) dy'd (*M*)

8th. Introducing my Son[290] to Kiss her hand, I afterwards discours'd of her having one of the Family of Hanover here, there occurring two reasons against it: one with respect to the Queen, least it should be the Occasion of disquiet between her, and that Family, there always being enough of Evil Instrument to act that Part. And if that Happen'd between Her Sister and Her, it was more likely to Happen between a more remote familly, and Her. Another Reason was with Respect to the Electors Family, Her People being mightily given to desire somewhat new, After knowing all that was to be known of them, their Inclinations might Crave after Another Viz the Pretender.

10th. To show her respect for the Duchess of Somerset, She askd if her complaints did not look like gravel; and if Tipping's Water[291] which I gave to Mrs. Foyston[292] so successfully was not suitable to the Duchess. If it was, that I might get a bottle of it for the Queen to give to the Duchess. She charging me not to say any thing of it, that She had it from me.

15th. I told the Queen what my son said of the Duke d'Aumonts Present of the Horses, that they should have been presented to her, when they first come over, and not after He had Us'd them.

20th. I told Her Peoples Objection against Her Speech,[293] for not having said one word of the Family of Hanover in it, and that the Nobility were Offended at being call'd from their differing from the Ministry, Factious. She said she meant All Her Subjects.

22nd. I hopd that now Peace was made, my Lord Oxford would keep Her in Constant Ease. She said He was Crazy,[294] and that if any thing happend to him, She would have a great loss of him. She heard there were some Whig Lords who heard, and liked the Thanksgiving Sermon, and said it was no Party One.

27th. She said that Mr. Hambden[295] came only to see, if she was Ill, and once a long time ago he had been with Her, and said, that might be the Reason the Examiner took Notice of it.

August 1st. Visiting the Queen, Lady Massam in a great Passion of Crying, in the Queens Hearing, and scolding at Mrs. Foyston and Mrs. Smith,[296] least they had thrown her Child down in the Queens room on purpose. I took notice of my Lady Massams Passion as unsuitable to the Queens Temper, and of the Duchess of Somerset's more Suitable, to which she reply'd. Yes by farr, but Suitable to Her natural goodness made an Excuse for my Lady Massams loud Passion, because the Child had been lately ill, and She was afraid of any hurt to come to it, mentioning from Hence, that to Calm dispositions a Suitable Friendship was the next to the Sensible Favour of God.

5th. She went to Windsor.

10th. Visiting the Queen at Hampton Court, Discours'd about the Adress to demolish Dunkirk;[297] and the book call'd the History of the Parliament,[298] telling Her how it look'd well in Her Majesty, to know such things, in Order to know the Mind of Her People, but Still I found that Repuls'd, by telling Her it was Party and Faction that was discontented, and not the Body of the Nation.

13th. Visiting Lord Cowper, he said that the first Sessions it was told that the Warr with Spain must be continu'd, to Stroak us, As they begin to tame a Wanton Horse: For at that time, what was Said in the Second Sessions would not have been borne; Viz: that the Power must be Ballanc'd, and that it was not safe to have the Emperour, King of Spain.[299] The Second Session a Treaty of Peace must be set on foot; and the third, it must be read, and Approv'd.

21st. Visiting the Queen at Windsor, Discours'd the Affair of Lady Mary,[300] and what Lord Oxford said. She ask'd me what they talk'd about the Changes.[301] I told Her they were so busy about the Elections, that they talk'd of Nothing Else.[302] And desir'd me to say nothing of the Duchess of Somerset's being gone to Petwith, and said it must be so, sometimes, He will have it so.

September 18th. Little Opportunity, but convers'd with the Duchess of Somerset, telling Her, how I lov'd the Queen and thought on everything for Her Quiet, and amongst other things, that of Her being much[w] with the Queen, In which I knew Her Majesty took great delight. She told me she always weigh'd what was Her Duty; and that neither the Frowns, nor the Smiles of a Court, shoud hinder Her from doing that. She said she ow'd a Duty to the Duke, and her Family, and that all her Spare time, that she had from her duty to the Queen, she must use it that way. But to Spend all Her Time with the Queen, was impossible. I endeavour'd to Convince Her of Her Majestys Affectionateness to Her, from Her concern in going from Her, She says, that cannot be, if the Duke of Somerset be gone a forthnight to Newmarket, must I be con-

[w] much (*M*) well (*M*)

cern'd. To which I said the Parallell was not the same, For you have Pleasure when He is gone, in Children, Visiting etc, but She has Uneasiness, and feels the Advantage of having your Grace to Converse with.

October 16th. The Queen fine and Well.

30th. She ask'd me if there was any Confusion Yesterday, to which I said No.

November 12th. Mr. Caesar from Hanover, his Conversation, and Mine.

13th. I told the Queen, Mr. Caesar[303] was come to town, with which she seem'd well Pleas'd, but delay'd hearing.

26th. The Queen Well, and had no Opportunity of Converse.

December 12th. Visiting the Queen. Converse about Mr. Cesar, Lady Carmarthen,[304] and Mrs. Donnellens letter.[305]

25th. Call'd to Windsor upon the Queens Illness.[306]

1714.

To February 17th. On which Day She came to Town. No opportunity of Private Discourse, the rest of the Phisitians generally going in with me, and at that time upon going in alone, Health seem'd the properest subject for discourse; That Evening Visiting Her she told me they pressd Her to Steel,[307] and desir'd me to consider of it, for Her dependance was on my Judgement.

25th. Asking if my Lord Cowper shoud wait upon her she answerd, Not too soon. I further Address'd my self thus. Madam I hope I have given Your Majesty no Offence, by what I have either said, or done, ever since I had the Honour to attend Your Majesty, as your Phisitian. If I have, its an Errour in my Judgement, and not in my Will. For my Aim in everything, has been, to keep Your mind quiet, and You thereby in Health, to keep you in the Affections of the People, and that every One may speak honourably of You. The reason why I mention this to your Majesty is, because I see some danger, in Staying long with Your Majesty, both of Disquiet to You, and making me the object of suspicion and Malice, and so of Hindering me, of serving Your Majesty as I have done. I'll therefore be Cautious till some time is over, To which She reply'd She could not but be satisfy'd with every thing I did, because I could have no End of my own, but only her Health, and Quiet, and said she lik'd my present Caution; I imagine the Differences among the Ministers were then rising to a Height,[308] and so rais'd more a Jelousie of any body that stay'd long with the Queen.

March 2nd. Visiting Lord Cowper after his being with the Queen, he told me, that in Conversation with Her, Her greatest concern seem'd to be, least any of the House of Hanover should come over, as undoubtedly had been suggested to Her.

April 7th. She was extreamly griev'd about the Talk of some of the Family of Hanover coming Over[309] and the

8th. 8th. her saying she would give any Security for the Succession if they would not let any of that Family come Over was the Occasion of their Acting thus.

12th. I express'd my Uneasiness at coming so seldom, Dr. Arburthnot having proposed April 9th. that Each Phisitian shoud only come, one a day, in his Own turn, which caus'd intermission of days in Attendance.

20th. In discourse presum'd to return to my former way of Conversation and then Vindicated my Lord Cowper, from having any Hand in the Duke of Cambridges calling for Writt.[310] And that he said he woud not have been for it without Convincing the Queen of the reasonableness of it.

23rd. Visiting Lord Cowper he desir'd me to suggest to the Queen that it would be better by farr not to mention the Treaty of Commerce. And it would give quiet to the People but Visiting the Queen the 23rd. I had no opportunity.

28th. She told me she did not believe the Duke of Cambridge woud come, and if He did his hot temper he was said to have woud Injure him.

May 6th. Visiting the Queen in discourse I ask'd if she knew Stinkins,[311] she answered short saying do you know him, to which I answered that he had been my acquaintance these 20 years. I ask'd if she knew Schullenburg.[312] She said Yes.

7th. A new Illness returning[313] my Mouth was stop'd, probably about Family of Hanover coming to Britain.

27th. Visiting the Palatine[314] he had call'd the Treasurer from the Queen, and shew'd him Burgs[315] letter, assuring that the Duke woud not come over. Lord Oxford laughed at what was mention'd in the letter about the Queen, if she was for the Pretender, and approv'd the Palatines saying that the way to maintain a Friendship, between the two Courts, was, by the Hanover Court's sending over hither a Minister, whom this Court liked and approv'd of and nam'd Burg. Oxford approv'd of him, and said he would write to the Electour, and also said that what was write of the

Character of Plimpton[316] was right, for he was as the letter said, and Oxfords endeavours woud be to remove some of the Court of Hanover. He told him that the letters of the 19th. to the Queen, said That the Elector had not as yet seen Schutz[317] Tho' all the Whigs said Otherwise; So that by Burgs being here, and the Palatine in Friendship with him, I shall be able to find out if the Queen be for the Pretender.

28th. The Palatine told me, that Oxford had a letter from Princess Sophia, The Elector, and Electoral Prince, and that in his reading the letter where 1200 men coud come up to London *and take it*, he said England had been often taken, and that it was always when there was a Standing Army that the Queen was intirely therein, and that he had agreed to write that Burg shoud come Over.

29th. The Palatine told me, that Oxford Laid the letter before the Queen to let her see it was not compliments to Tom Harley.[318]

June 1st. Visiting the Queen I ask'd if she saw the Palatines letter, she said Yes, and ask'd if I had seen it. For seing Her Ill, and supposing Her concern to have a hand in it, I ask'd for it that morning she was taken Ill. I said I hop'd she would give Credit to what my Lord Clarendon[319] wrote, and thereby be made Easy if this letter did not do it, asking if she had any commands for me, or if I had done aright. To which she said Yes, but pray'd me to go no further in it.

2nd. Visiting Lord Cowper, he gave me two signs of Bulingbrokes gaining Ground. The first was my Lord Clarendons going over to the Court of Hanover, the 2nd. was his obtaining for his Brother the Embassy, with £600 for his Equipage and £2000 a year Allowance.[320]

5th. Visiting the Queen and asking leave for my Lord Cowper to wait upon Her, she seem'd to Shift it of, from Outward Influence, for she always before shewd a ready Inclination to it, tho' a Prudent regard as to the time of his coming; She saying My Lord us'd to come at his going out of town, and return to it; and his going out of town being so near, the properest time would be before he went out of Town. I ask'd her if Princess Sophia's Death[321] added any thing to Her quiet or disquiet, To which she said, that Princess Sophia was Chipping-Porridge[322] it would neither give more Ease, nor more uneasiness.

9th. Visiting Her Majesty at St. James and she asking if any thing troubled me, I took that opportunity to Repeat to Her my Advice against Disquiet, telling her not only from my Experience in Others but in my self, how dangerous disquiet was in the Gout, to Cause Sudden dangerous Translations. For since I had waited upon Her Majesty, upon reading a letter with the Account of my Mothers Death,[323] and her last declaration of my Duty, and leaving Her last blessing upon that Account, in less than a Quarter of an hour, there happen'd Such a Translation of a Gouty pain, from my left foot to my Stomach; with the Violence of which, so dispiriting and throwing me into Cold Sweats that I thought I should have dy'd, if means had not imediately succeeded; Not knowing what was to happen to Her, Such Cautions to Her, and all about Her, having been my habitual Custom.

15th. Visiting Lord Cowper. Said that all teaching English, and writing was allow'd, that Under this they would Teach other things,[324] that in the Act of Uniformity these very things now allow'd were prohibited, so that by this Allowance the Act of Uniformity was weaken'd. That Oxford had ruin'd his own business by being against the Bill. That the Duke shoud not come over 'till the Queen was in Danger.[325]

21st. Discours'd only of Steel,[326] it having been propos'd.

25th. I told her that some reported that my Lord Oxford would be out, and others that Bolingbroke woud be out.

29th. She enquiring with some seeming Concern ask'd me How I did, because Mrs. Danvers told Her I had been Suddenly Affected with a dimness in my Sight, in gratitude to which I repeated my Advice to Her to Shun Disquiet at least the Ill Effects of it. She said, As much as she could.

July 3rd. Visiting the Queen I acquainted Her of a Charitable Petition concerning a Pension of a Ladies in Scotland.[327]

6th. Visiting Lord Cowper he told me that to day it had been found out in the house that Mr. Arthur More had Authority tó make the Peace, and at the same time had a Promise from the King of Spain, to be one of his Commissioners; but that Mr. Orry[328] had writt, that his Commission was not to be sign'd till the three Articles on which all hinged, were Sign'd here etc.

7th In Converse with the Queen, I told her I had a letter from the Palatine, telling me, he had wrote to my Lord Oxford, a further account of the Assurance of the Dukes not coming over, on purpose to quiet the Queens mind; But that my Lord Oxford never giving any return to that Burg desisted from writing any more. Upon which I said, I wonderd that my Lord neglected writing an Answer, for by that Means her Majesty wanted the Knowledge of things, which Perhaps might have given her Pleasure. To which she said, I know not how he comes to do so, but I'll convey an answer to Burg by some other hand. Which confirm'd of my Lord Oxfords declining in the Queens Favour and Trust Else he would have been the Person she would have spoke to. She said that if the Money Bill Pass'd, she would go to the House the next day.[329]

9th. Lord Cowper acquainted me with the Queens Answer to the Houses Address that her part of the Money might be appropriated to the South Sea; Viz; that she had the greatest Regard, for the Opinion of the Lords and she would do with her Own, what she Pleas'd.[330] How it provok'd the House to a laughter: My Lord Anglesy[331] and Lord Wharton[332] to hot Speeches, My Lord Cowper Arguing against its being printed, so that the World might not know any difference between the Queen, and the House.

12th. Visiting the Queen she was indispos'd at Her Stomach, suppos'd to be from something she eated the night before. But however that might be Disquiet concurr'd from the Accounts were given Her, of the Hot speeches that were made Upon Her Answer to the Address of the House about the South Sea. For upon my asking when Lord Cowper shoud wait upon Her, before he went out of Town she answer'd me with much inward concern thus; I thought he had been so angry with me, that he would not have seen me, some Person or other representing His Carriage worse than the rest. For upon my telling Her, that I had it from his Own mouth, that his Speech reffer'd Only to hinder the printing her Majestys Answer, so that the world might not be privy to any Heat between the Queen and Parliament she answer'd that she had heard of my Lord Cowpers carriage from *an Indifferent Hand.*[x][333] From whence it plainly appears, that false Insinuations, and Misrepresentations (from whom they come is best know[n] to their own Consciences) of Persons, and Things Misled the Queens Judgement, Impress'd Her against Persons, and made Her Yeild to the Direction of Others. For by Management few were admitted to

[x] Mr Coke Vicechamberlain (*Marginal note* (*M*))

give Her a Contrary Account to what was habitually Sounding In Her Ears. And if at any time it was done, she either was under an Awe of mentioning it, least the Person who was so kind to Suggest to Her had been injur'd by if she did mention it, the Influence of the Persons who gave answers to what she might Mention, was more than that of the Person who in kindness suggested any Thing to Her, Else putting Confusion, and Commotion among the Persons then Trusted, which she hated as any Mortal Poyson, or Stopping Her proceedings in Business were Motives to make her Yeild.

15th. In discourse with the Queen only read Lord Cowpers letter of Excuse for not waiting upon Her, before He went out of town. Viz the Sudden Illness of his Children as Also,[334] the Palatine's letter to me, wherein he assur'd me of the little Occasion the Queen had to fear the Duke's coming Over. His letters reaching the Electours Own hands, and with Acceptance, so that his returns from thence may be depended Upon.

19th. In discourse with the Queen, she only mention'd that of the Duke's coming Over.[335]

23rd. Visiting the Queen was concern'd at Lady Massams Waiting least it had hinderd me of time with the Queen. But Lady Massam with great Civility calling me in to her, and telling me, that as my Lord Oxford, and old Mrs. Foley[336] had abus'd me, so they would abuse Her, concerning Lord Massams having a Reversion after Lord Finch's death,[337] which he had desir'd Lady Massam to ask for him from the Queen when he was Secretary. Which her Majesty did not give him 'till he was Treasurer. But Upon his Sons being marry'd to the Duke of Newcastles Daughter, he asking the Title of Duke of Newcastle and Her Majesty refusing it, with Seeming Resentment at it,[338] Desir'd the Queen to give the Reversion to Lord Massam; his Family being Sufficiently Provided for. But tho' Lady Massam refus'd it, yet upon his repeated denial of accepting it, the Queen bestow'd it upon Her. She telling me at the same time, that he had never Acted Right in the Queens Affairs since his being refus'd the Title of Duke of Newcastle. Upon this Conversation, I told Lady Massam, that I was to mention a Charitable Pension for a Lady in Scotland, but I was so bashfull in taking Notice of any such thing to the Queen, that it would take me time, before I could bring it out. This I said as an excuse for Staying with the Queen. Coming in to Her, I told Her of Lady Massams Civility, and my Contrivance of an Excuse to stay without Suspition of me, or Disquiet to Her Self, and therefore, that I might not lye, she'd be forc'd to repeat my Charitable Petition for the Scots Lady, asking what I should say to Lady Massam about it, she Order'd me to Say, that when my Lord Marr mention'd it to Her, she would do it. She desir'd me at the Same time to write to *Bourg* to come to town, she thought to have conveyd what matter to write, but she had none to trust, she would give me a proof of what Trust she put in me. For she found that the many things which she had suggested were true, particularly her Subjects Fear that she was for the Pretender. When she had been talkd of to be at the head of the Protestant Religion, Shoud she be an Instrument of Ruining it in Her Own Kingdoms. But she had been dealt insincerely with, and teaz'd to do many Things against her own Inclination, particularly That, of turning my Lord Godolphin Out;[339] remembring me of what I had said to Her, Viz: that I told my Lord Oxford that People said he would learn Her to Equivocate, and Mrs. Harley at my Own house that Mr. Harley[y] needed not be afraid of the Malice of the Whig Ministry, If he was a Sincere man, and minded sincerely the good of the Nation, but that if He did not Act with Integrity, that it would not be in the Queens Power to Save him. As also my Lord Cowpers Answer to Her, desiring him to Stay In, by me, That he saw so much Tricking and Shuffling that he could not with Ease of Mind join in it. This discourse melted me to that Degree, that Lady Massam was Surpris'd to see me come out with Such a Violent heat, and ask'd me if the Queen had refus'd the Petition, to which I answered No, but my bashfullness always makes me come out from the Queen in such a Colour. But it was from resentment at those, whoever they were, who had brought Her to that Distress of Mind, and from the pleasure I had to see Her, trust in me as a reward of my faithfullness as her Phisitian, and my Unbiass'd regard to Her, as Her Subject.

27th. Visiting the Palatine in my way to the Queen at Kensignton, he gave me a Copy of a letter of the Electors to Bourg, in which he express'd his Satisfaction with Bourgs Correspondance letters, and the Inteligence which he gave, desiring him to Comunicate

[y] Lord Oxford (*Marginal note* (*M*))

any thing Material, that was further Comunicated to him. Then in converse with the Queen I showd Her this letter, as a proof to her, that what the Palatine wrote, was from the Electors own hands without any Ones knowledge, but Bourgs, and that what came from Bourg she might depend upon as truth, to Quiet her Mind, the Duke of Cambridge, not being to come Over. But she said that gave her no Uneasiness Now. She asking if I could trust the Palatine because he was a Roman Catholic. To which I answerd that I did not know any thing Ill of him, Nor no other way at Present of conveying, any thing she would say, with that Privacy and Success. Upon which she said that imediately she desir'd he should write over, so that it might come to the Electour by the hand of Bourg, that the Changes she was about to make, shoud not injure him, nor lessen Her friendship to him unless he was the Cause of it himself, by Personal Ingratitude, and that if he would write to Her upon this Her Profession of friendship, she would Immediately answer it with Her own hand, without the knowledge of any of Her Ministry, and desir'd that his writing might be without the knowledge of any of his. For most of them sought themselves, they had neither regarded Her health, Her life, nor Her peace. But at the Same time askd me if I could find no Excuse to go to Hanover without Peoples Suspicion of being sent. To which I said, Yes, by removing my Son from Oxford, and settling him at Leyden or Utrecht, I could have the Excuse of going Over with him, having now No familly, and by asking Openly Her Majestys leave to see Hanover. For as I never had to do with any body but her self, she being Easie and pleas'd with me, I was above the disregard of any body Else, having always hitherto carry'd in that Manner. And Then asking Her of my Errand thither she told me it was to Settle a Sincere Friendship with the Elector, and that all occasions of Jealousie might be remov'd, and in Such a way, as would give Her Self least disquiet. Her own letter, and what History I could give him of my self would Secure me of his Confidence to Open to me and to Write to Her. For He was to ask leave to come Over to pay a Visit to Her for three or four weeks by which Means he would have entire Satisfaction, and She Quiet, she resolving to put it upon him to make Changes. This Confidence affected me, even to Tears; and returning from Her, had the first part of This writt over by the Palatine to the

Electour by Bourg that night, as the first Step. The other being to be known to none but her Majesty, the Elector, and my self. These letters containing the first part of what is said came to the Electors hands, but sudden Death coming in prevented Her going on, for she told me Lord Oxford would be out that night, and upon Telling Her that Bolingbroke was said to get the Staff, she said No as also my telling Her that Persons said the Reason why my Lord Oxford was to be out, was because he had hinder'd Her Majesty from giving Grants to Lady Massam, to which she answerd that if he said so, he was very ungrateful to Lady Massam.

29th. Being call'd in the Morning to meet the Other Phisitians, she had a trembling in Her hands, a Pain and Heat in Her head, with Sleepiness, and a little bleeding at the Nose etc. as mention'd in the foregoing History, and in three days Death Succeeded, the Preventer of all future projected Thoughts.

By this it plainly appears, that from Her Majestys Infancy, to Her Death, she had no Complaint, but what was the Common Effect of a Sharpness in her blood, discharging Outward, the Common forms of Ails, to preserve Her Constitution, 'till within these few years, a succession of disquiets happen'd, which weakend Her Nerves; and prepar'd them for receiving a translation of this Sharpness, threatning first, to discharge on the foot, and knee, in the Form of the Gout, but her Spirits being thus weakly at that time, it would not perform: it translated upwards upon the Nerves, and Brain. So that all the Stories of Her Majestys supposed Ails, and complaints *were utterly false* and the Effect of a lying Corrupt Spirit, rais'd up as Dr. Bradford says in his sermon Out of the Infernal Pitt, from the Rage of Party Conversation, which is so prevalent, that it not only makes Persons hear reproaches, with an Open Ear, and greediness ready to believe and hasty to tell it again with the Device of Satan, as if they were concern'd for the Person, when they are pleas'd with the reproach of them but which is still more surprising, ever unwilling to be inform'd, and to believe the Contrary, Yea sooner give Credit to an Ill person telling the reproach, than to a known good person, contradicting it. Yea the Spirit leads them further Still, to add Another Sin to that of reproaching, boldly to affirm, that they knew it to be true, when they knew it from no where Else but the mouth of the Corrupt reproacher. How many have mention'd to me a

Monstrous description of Dropsycal Swelling, of her Majestys limbs and Elsewhere, when I have been Vindicating Her Constitution, as without any Tendency to it, and Tho' Her Royal Body, when Dissected declar'd the truth thereof,[340] yet the reproachers, hold on, their Breathing out their Venom, by saying she was tapp'd the night before, I hope I may with the same Justice Vindicate Her Mind, and Abstracting it from Impositions upon Her, and Misguidings of Others. She had a Mind, and Inclinations therein Pious towards God, and to make all Her Subjects Easie, instead of reproaching them, as they have done Her. I have stood in Amaze My Self, to hear Her make excuses for Others. And for Civility and good breeding she bears the Character, among Her Greatest Enemys. A mind Pious towards God, willing to please all its fellow Creatures, calm and Courteous in Conversation, unwilling to believe Reproaches of others, or to cast them Upon Any; Dutyfull to A Husband, and one of the best Mistresses to Servants; Such a Mind upon the Throne, dos it not Resemble the Sun in the Firmament. But when a Cloud is near it or before it, how is its beautiful Aspect and its desirable Influence, Chang'd and lessen'd, while the Sun, it its self is the Same. In like manner, while a Cloud of Persons stands between and near Her Majesty thus describ'd, and her People, how dos it not alter her aspect, and benign Influence, Upon Her People, while She in her own Mind is the Same. Can you read the last part of this, of the Queen Acting from her Own Mind and Inclination, free from Clouds of Ministry advising between Her, and Her People, and will you Impute past Accidents to a Corrupt mind in the Queen. She in Her Self, and from Her self contriving the removing the Jealousies of Her People, and the Clouds Her Ministry had cast upon Her, the Securing the Protestant Religion, in the Protestant Succession, and the Retrieving Her Own honour, by Showing Her Self Naturally as She is. Will you therefore go on to say that in Her own Mind, and of Her self, she was the Betrayer of your libertys, and the Destroyer, of the Protestant Religion, by too great a Regard for the Pretender. Lett Others thunder and reproach as much as they will, I shall always retain a good Opinion, till I see higher proof against it. Turn therefore Upon Your Clouds, Scatter them, and the Sun will appear in its brightness, and let His Majesty who Succeeds be guided from Himself, who seems to have such Advantages of mind, as to Guide and Protect his People, with gainfull and pleasant Influences. And then He'll escape the reproach of his Predecessor by casting of the Old Advisers, and Regulating the new according to His own Mind.

NOTES

1. William, Duke of Gloucester (1689–1700) died in July 1700 a few days after his eleventh birthday. Anne 'bore his death with a resignation and piety that were indeed very singular' (Burnet, iv. 452).

2. Mary (1662–94) was, like Anne, the daughter of James II by his first wife Anne Hyde. For the estrangement between the two sisters, resulting from disagreements over Anne's accommodation, allowance, and above all her continued friendship with the Churchills after Marlborough's disgrace in 1692, see *Conduct*, pp. 24–109.

3. Attempts at an incorporating Union with Scotland had been made ever since the accession of James VI and I in 1603 had joined the two crowns. Abortive efforts had been made by Cromwell, Charles II, William III, and even by Anne during the first year of her reign. Union was finally achieved on 6 Mar. 1707 when Anne gave her assent to the union bill (Luttrell, vi. 145–6). Her pleasure at this success is reputed to have led her to say that 'The union with Scotland is the happiness of my reign' (Strickland, viii. 270).

4. Although Anne was pleased with the news of Blenheim in 1704 and Ramillies in 1706 she is alleged to have remarked 'Oh Lord, when will all this dreadful bloodshed cease' on learning about the battle of Oudenarde in 1708 (quoted in David Green, *Queen Anne*, p. 191).

5. Anne's popular reputation for piety can be gauged from the addresses presented to her in 1710. The Warwickshire address referred to her 'exemplary piety', and in the Radnorshire address she was called 'the most pious and best of princes' (*A Collection of the Addresses which have been presented to the Queen* (1710), pp. 6, 9). The most practical expression of her piety was, of course, the grant of Queen Anne's Bounty to augment the stipends of poor clergymen.

6. The death of her husband Prince George of Denmark on 28 Oct. 1708 considerably distracted Anne. The Paymaster General, James Brydges, was struck by her 'agonies of grief', while even the Duchess of Marlborough conceded that 'she was certainly more concerned for him than she was for the fate of Gloucester' (Huntington Library, Stowe MSS. 57. ii. 99: *Priv. Corr.* i. 416).

7. Another possible motive besides his alleged ignorance for not wanting to enlarge on the effect of Sarah's tantrums on Anne is that Hamilton was anxious to minimize the bad effects on the Queen of his Whig acquaintances, and to stress those of his Tory enemies. The Duchess of Marlborough's 'ungovernable rage', according to Swift, 'had long alienated her sovereign's mind, before it appeared to the world' (*The History of the Four Last Years of the Queen* (1758), p. 17). Anne's private dissatisfaction with Sarah dated from 1705 (Churchill, *Marlborough*, iii. 265). It became open on Harley's fall in 1708, which made Anne ill, Sir John Cropley reporting to the Earl of Shaftesbury on 5 Feb. 'The Q is not well, grieves much, has had the gout in her stomach' (PRO 30/24/21/145 and see 150).

8. Luttrell noted on 6 Dec. 1709 'Her majestie being somewhat indisposed with the gout, went not to chappel on Sunday last' [4 Dec.] (Luttrell, vi. 519).

9. Sidney, first Earl of Godolphin (1645–1712), Anne's treasurer since 1702, was off-putting in his appearance and manner. Macky noted that Godolphin 'hath an admirable, clear understanding, of slow speech, with an awful, serious Deportment; does more than he promises; an Enemy to Flattery, Shew and Violence; of very hard Access; but that being equally denied to all Degrees of People, makes it supportable; of a low stature; thin, with a very black and stern countenance' (*Memoirs of the Secret Services of John Macky, Esq.* [Roxburgh Club, 1895], p. 43).

10. 'The next specific I esteem to be that little insect called *Millepedes*: the powder whereof, made up into little balls with fresh butter, I never knew fail of curing any sore throat . . . and should be very tedious if I should tell here, how much the use of it has been extolled by several within my knowledge, upon the admirable effects, for the eyes, the scurvy, and the gout . . .' (Sir W. Temple, 'Of Health and Long Life', *Works* (Edinburgh, 1754), ii. 423).

11. It was characteristic of Godolphin to use an earthy metaphor. He once said that 'a discreet clergyman is almost as rare as a black swan', and often compared his lot with that of a galley slave (HMC *Bath*, i. 63: BM Loan 29/64).

12. Others were surprised how accommodating Godolphin could be once they had penetrated his initial reserve. Thus Sir John Cropley wrote to his patron Lord Shaftesbury, within days of his first interview with him to request a favour, 'All allow no minister did ever execute his promises speedilyer [*sic*] or handsomelyer than my lord Treasurer' (PRO/30/24/20/141 i).

13. Godolphin is here referring not to the Privy Council but to the Cabinet Council. Ministers who attended it called themselves 'the Lords of the Committee' when the Queen was not present (J. H. Plumb, 'The organisation of the Cabinet in the reign of Queen Anne', *Transactions of the Royal Historical Society*, 5th ser., 7 (1957), 137–57).

14. Several places were vacant at this time, including the treasurership of the Navy, which went to Robert Walpole on 14 Jan. (Luttrell, vi. 534). But the business Anne most probably anticipated was that concerning the disposal of the posts of constable of the Tower and colonel of a regiment of dragoons, both vacant by the death of the Earl of Essex that very day (ibid.).

15. John Hill (d. 1735) was the brother of Abigail, the bedchamberwoman who had replaced the Duchess of Marlborough as Anne's favourite. Both were cousins of the Duchess, and had been introduced into the royal service by her. John had been made a page to the Queen. He had also followed a military career, commanding a brigade at the battle of Almanza in 1707 and being wounded at Mons in 1709. Anne's intention to bestow a vacant regiment upon him in January caused a major political crisis, at the height of which the Duke of Marlborough came very close to resigning. The Duke retired to Windsor Lodge, from which he protested against 'the malice of a bed-chamber woman'. He was eventually persuaded to return to London on 23 Jan., and saw Anne on the 24th. The upshot was a compromise, 'neither Meredith, proposed by the Duke to succeed to my Ld Essex's Regmt of Dragoons, nor Hill, to whom the Queen had given it, should have it,

but that it should be given to Sr. Richard Temple . . . and that Hill should have a pension of £1000 per annum out of the Post Office for the Queen's Life' ('Earl Coningsbie's History of Parties presented to King George the first' *Archaeologia*, 38 (1860), 11. See also Coxe, the *Conduct*, and the Mainwaring letters in Blenheim MSS. E. 25).

16. A vote to address the Queen to remove Abigail from her service was to be introduced into the Commons on 23 Jan. (Boyer, ix. 229). The idea apparently originated with Arthur Mainwaring (1668–1712), who was M.P. for Preston, auditor of the imprests, and the Duchess of Marlborough's private secretary. The measure was adopted by Sunderland and the extreme supporters of Marlborough's stand against the Queen to force Anne to agree with the Duke's demands (Blenheim MSS. E. 27; Arthur Mainwaring to the Duchess of Marlborough, 'Monday afternoon' [? 23 January 1710]). The proposal thoroughly alarmed the Queen who 'sent for several persons of both Houses in her service, declared with great spirit and courage against it . . . among these is said to be . . . Mainwaring, to whom she spoke very plain' (Leicestershire RO, Finch MSS., DG. 7, bdle. 23: newsletter, 28 Jan. 1709/10).

17. Henry Sacheverell (1674–1724) fellow of Magdalen College, Oxford, and chaplain of St. Saviour's, Southwark, underwent trial before the House of Lords, on charges of impeachment brought against him by the House of Commons, from 27 Feb. to 23 Mar. 1710. The charges arose out of sermons delivered by him at the Derby assizes in August 1709 and in St. Paul's cathedral on 5 Nov. 1709, the Commons alleging that in them he had impugned the Revolution Settlement, attacked the Toleration Act, and insinuated that both Church and State were in danger under her Majesty's administration. See Holmes, *Trial*.

18. These divisions of opinion were to appear openly in the debate in the House of Lords on 21 Mar. 1709 about what censure to pass on Sacheverell. See Holmes, *Trial*, pp. 228–9.

19. Apparently Anne changed her mind in the course of the trial, for initially she told Burnet 'that it was a bad sermon, and that he deserved well to be punished for it' (Burnet, v. 446). Later the Marquis of Kent discovered that 'she thought the Commons had reason to be sattisfied that they had made their allegations good, and the mildest punishment inflicted upon the Doctor she thought the best' (*Wentworth Papers*, p. 146).

20. For the 'riot night' of 1 Mar. 1710 on which six dissenting meeting-houses were sacked, and troops had to be called out to deal with five mobs, as a result of which 105 people were committed to gaol, see Holmes, *Trial*, pp. 156–76.

21. i.e. the person who recommended the insertion in the Queen's speech to parliament at the close of the session on 5 Apr. It was almost certainly Lord Cowper, with whom Hamilton was intimately acquainted (see Introduction, p. xvii). Cowper offered similar advice about the clergy to George I (Lord Campbell, *Lives of the Lord Chancellors* (1846), iv. 429).

22. Hamilton again seems reluctant to censure the Duchess of Marlborough, (cf. p. 70 n. 7). Sarah had seen the Queen on 3 Apr. to request an interview, which had been arranged for 6 p.m. on the 4th, the day Hamilton records his own conversation with the Queen here. In fact Anne postponed the meeting, writing to the Duchess 'to lay before her in writing whatever I had to say, and to gratify myself in going into the country as soon as

I could' (*Conduct*, p. 237). Instead Sarah persisted in seeing her, and on 6 Apr. there occurred the stormy confrontation which ended their long acquaintance (ibid., pp. 238–44; *Priv. Corr.* i. 295–9).

23. Between 4 and 19 Apr., a period when there is a gap in the diary, the Queen removed the Marquis of Kent from the post of Lord Chamberlain and replaced him, at Harley's instigation, with the Duke of Shrewsbury on 14 Apr. (Luttrell, vi. 570). Charles Talbot, first Duke of Shrewsbury (1660–1718) had played a leading role in the Revolution of 1688 and in William's reign was Secretary of State from 1689 to 1690 and again from 1694 to 1700. Implicated in the Jacobite intrigues of 1696, however, he had withdrawn from ministerial activity before he obtained William's permission to go abroad in 1700. He spent the next six years on the continent, mostly in Italy. On his return in 1706 he was cold-shouldered by his former Whig colleagues, and gravitated into Harley's circle. By 1709 Harley had obtained audiences with the Queen for him (Coxe, iii. 57–60). He opposed the government in the Sacheverell trial, voting the Doctor not guilty in the division on 20 Mar. 1710 (Holmes, *Trial*, p. 284).

24. The appointment of Shrewsbury was unexpected in view of the Queen's speech on the proroguing of parliament on 5 Apr., which had reassured the Whigs (Cobbett, *Parliamentary History*, vi. 897–8; Burnet, v. 451). It initially 'gave a great alarm; for it was upon that concluded that a total change of the ministry would quickly follow' (Burnet, v. 454). However, the introduction into the government of a man with a Whiggish past meant that his elevation was not viewed with as much alarm as the appointment of a high-church man would have produced, and Shrewsbury managed to reassure the Whigs that he had not changed (ibid., p. 440; Coxe, iii. 67–70).

25. The Marquis of Kent, had owed his post to the Duchess of Marlborough (Holmes, p. 211 and note). His replacement, therefore, was a slight against her, if only indirectly.

26. See Introduction, p. xxxiv.

27. See Introduction, p. xxxv n. 92.

28. For a discussion of the credit crisis aggravated by the ministerial changes of 1710 see B. W. Hill 'The change of government and the "loss of the City", 1710–11', *Economic History Review*, 24 (1971), 395–413.

29. Godolphin's son Francis, Viscount Rialton (1678–1766) married Henrietta Churchill, the Marlboroughs' eldest daughter, in 1698.

30. The team of Lord Treasurer and Captain General was so united that historians are generally correct in referring to the government in the years 1702 to 1710 as the Marlborough–Godolphin ministry. Political tensions, however, occasionally subjected the partnership to considerable strain. The crisis over Harley's fall in February 1708, for instance, produced a rift between the two friends which almost led Marlborough to throw in his lot with Harley and part company with Godolphin (G. S. Holmes and W. A. Speck, 'The fall of Harley in 1708 reconsidered', *English Historical Review*, 80 (1965), 687–9). Anne was therefore not entirely guilty of wishful thinking when speculating on the possibility of detaching Godolphin from the Duchess.

31. The latest negotiations between France and the partners of the Grand Alliance opened

in Gertruydenburgh in mid March (Luttrell, vi. 557). Godolphin feared that ministerial changes in England would either lead Louis XIV to drag out the negotiations in hopes of a better deal from the new ministers, or incline the allies to compromise in order to reach an early settlement. Louis in fact called off the negotiations in July. Although they broke down because he refused to agree to assist the allies to remove his grandson from the throne of Spain, the Whigs were convinced that the triumph of high-church Toryism in England had encouraged his move (*The French king's reasons against peace*, 1710; cf. Burnet, vi. 7: Hardwicke's note). They disapproved of the opening of discussions between Harley's agent the Earl of Jersey and the Abbé Gaultier in July 1710.

32. ? J. Beck (See entry for 10 Jan. 1712, p. 37; 2 Jan. 1713, p. 48. He has not been identified).

33. Abigail was not in fact preferred until January 1711, when she succeeded the Duchess of Marlborough as keeper of the privy purse (Luttrell, vi. 680).

34. Charles Spencer, 3rd Earl of Sunderland (1674–1722) was Marlborough's son-in-law and the junior Lord of the Whig Junto. He was dismissed from his post of Secretary of State not on 15 June but on 14 June 1710 (Luttrell, vi. 594). His removal had been held up for some time until Harley and the Queen could settle on the right replacement (Burnet, vi. 9: Dartmouth's note). Boyer suggests that the occasion of his fall was Sunderland's part as 'chief promoter of the design to deprive the queen of Mrs. Masham's attendance' (Boyer, *Annals*, ix. 230: cf. p. 72 n. 16).

35. See Introduction, p. xxxv ff.

36. Sarah later put the figure at 'near £90,000' (*Conduct*, p. 279).

37. Anne had made a similar statement the previous night when she saw a delegation of the Governor, Deputy-Governor, and two Directors of the Bank of England. In view of the fact that Anne was virtually called a liar when shortly afterwards she dismissed Godolphin (see p. 75 n. 49), it is interesting to note Boyer's record of the words used by Anne at this interview: 'She had not yet determin'd to make any other changes; and whenever she should, she would take care that the Publick Credit might not be injur'd thereby' (Boyer, *Annals*, ix. 232).

38. It is significant that the Queen left this option open, in view of the current notion that her reassurance to the Bankers meant 'that there will be no danger of dissolution' (*Huntington Lib. Quart.*, 3 (1940), 230).

39. The entry for 15 June from here to the end represents Hamilton's hindsight and not his strictly contemporary observations. It is probably true that at that time Anne did not desire further changes. What 'scheme' Harley had in mind is less easy to establish. The removal of Godolphin almost certainly featured in his plans from the beginning. Beyond this, however, and at this point, Harley probably did not want to go much further. For instance, his negotiations to retain Cowper as Lord Chancellor suggest that he wanted as few changes as necessary (see p. 81 n. 93).

40. Sir Richard Onslow (1654–1717) was one of the leading Country Whigs in the House of Commons (where he sat for Surrey from 1689 to 1710 and again from 1713 to 1716) until 1708 when he accepted the Court nomination to be Speaker in the 1708–10 parlia-

ment. He was admitted to the privy council on 17 June 1710 (Luttrell, vi. 595). Commenting on this two months later William Bromley observed to Dr. Charlett 'The taking him into the Council could not be at this time to prejudice his election' (Bod., Ballard MSS. 38, f. 150).

41. For the deputation from the Bank which waited on the Queen on 14 June see p. 74 n. 37.

42. Francis Eyles was one of the directors of the Bank of England who waited on the Queen on 14 June (Luttrell, vi. 594). In the event he did not stand for parliament, becoming instead sheriff of London and Middlesex on 28 Sept. (ibid., p. 634). His son John, however, successfully stood at Chippenham in the General Election (Holmes, p. 181).

43. 'On the day after Sunderland's dismissal the Bank . . . received from the Treasury a request for a routine loan of £120,000' (B. W. Hill, 'The change of government and the "loss of the City", 1710–11', p. 400). Godolphin must have been sent an unofficial notification of the Bank's attitude on the 17th, since it was not until 22 June that the Court of Directors considered the matter in the light of the views of those who had waited on the Queen, but refused this request.

44. i.e. Windsor Lodge, a house occupied by Sarah in her capacity as ranger of Windsor Forest, a post granted to her for life by the Queen, and therefore one which she retained when Anne removed her from all her other posts (Luttrell, vi. 680).

45. Presumably in her apartments at St. James's, since Marlborough house, which Sir Christopher Wren built for Sarah in Pall Mall, though commenced in 1709, was not ready until 1711 (David Green, *Queen Anne*, p. 210).

46. John Ward of Hackney was a leading City merchant, a director of the New East India Company from 1703 until its amalgamation with the Old in 1709, and a director of the Bank of England from 1698 to 1726, serving as Governor from 1701 to 1703. M.P. for Bletchingly from 1701 to 1708, London 1708–10, 1715–22, and Reigate from 1710 to 1713, where he was counted as a Tory (Luttrell, vi. 295) though he voted erratically and appears as a Whig in e.g. the Worsley list in Lincoln Record Office (published in the *History of Parliament 1715–1754*, ed. R. Sedgwick (1970), pp. 162–87).

47. Bank stock stood at 117¼ on 7 July, 115 on 19 July and 112¾ on 24 July. (Bod. Library, *Nichols Newspapers*, 17A).

48. Defoe had countered charges that credit depended upon the particular compositions of ministries or parliaments in *An Essay upon publick credit* (1710).

49. On 3 July Harley had written a memorandum preparatory to seeing the Queen, saying 'you must preserve your character and spirit and speak to lord Treasurer. Get quit of him' (BM Loan 29/10/19 quoted in B. W. Hill, 'The change of government and the "loss of the City" 1710–11', p. 401, note 3). Anne hesitated, apparently waiting a proper pretext. James Brydges put her resolution down to the Bank's unwillingness to lend any money, 'till her Majesty had made a further declaration that she intended no further changes, nor a Dissolution' (ibid., note 10).

50. Bank stock stood at 113 on 7 and 8 August, and fell to 108¾ between the 9th and the 11th (*British Mercury*, 7–11 Aug. 1710).

51. James Francis Edward (1688–1766) was the only son of James II and Mary of Modena. He had been taken to France during the Revolution, and was recognized as James III by Louis XIV on his father's death in 1701. He had other official titles, including the Chevalier de St. George, and, in 1712, the Duke of Gloucester (see p. 95 n. 229). He also had various nicknames, the most common being 'the Pretender' and 'Perkin'.

52. See p. 74 n. 37.

53. It is difficult to decide whether 'of late' refers to a pamphlet published after Anne's death, or is a strictly contemporary observation on the events of August 1710 which Hamilton has incorporated into later reflections. For a strictly contemporary assertion that Anne had broken her word see next note.

54. *Queries* was a half-sheet printed on both sides. It is reprinted in *Somers Tracts*, xii. 668–70. '[Erasmus] Lewis the undersecretary has taken up the woman that sells pamphlets at Charing-Cross for selling the *Queries*: examined her about the printer and author. She said she knew neither: she sold them in the way of her trade, and it was her livelihood... So he let her go again, and was as wise as before' (Blenheim MSS. E 27: Arthur Mainwaring to the Duchess of Marlborough 'Monday morning after eight o'clock' [25 Aug. 1710]).

55. Although Harley was merely made a member of the commission of the treasury which replaced Godolphin on 10 Aug. (at the head of which was Lord Poulet), being at the same time made Chancellor of the Exchequer (Luttrell, vi. 616), it was clear to contemporaries that he had really replaced Godolphin as prime minister (Holmes, p. 440).

56. Charles Seymour (1662–1748) sixth Duke of Somerset, had been made Master of the Horse at the Queen's accession in 1702. Although in the previous reign he had been a Tory, about 1701 he became a Whig (T. Forster, *Original letters of Locke, Algernon Sidney and lord Shaftesbury* (1833), p. 193). In 1710, however, he fell in with Harley's schemes, and intrigued against his Whig colleagues in the ministry until the dissolution of parliament (Coxe, iii. 26, 79–80, 97, 118).

57. Sarah continued to assert that Anne's letter of dismissal to Godolphin 'was sent by no worthier messenger than a man in livery, to be left with his lordship's porter' (*Conduct*, p. 260). Lord Dartmouth was scathing about this; 'The princess of Mindelheim [Sarah] says, the queen sent her letter for dismissing Godolphin from her service, by a livery man, to be left with his porter . . . The letter was sent by Mr. Smith, a particular friend of his own, who was then chancellor of the exchequer, and afterwards a teller for life, at his recommendation . . .' (Burnet, vi. 10, note). This conflict of witnesses is apparently resolved by Swift, who wrote to Archbishop King on 9 Sept. 'A Letter was sent him by the Groom of the Queen's Stables, to desire he would break his Staff, which would be the easiest Way, both to her Majesty and him. Mr. *Smith*, Chancellor of the Exchequer, happening to come in a little after, my Lord broke his Staff, and flung the Pieces in the Chimney, desiring Mr. *Smith* to be Witness that he had obeyed the Queen's Commands, and sent him to the Queen with a Letter, and a Message, which Mr. *Smith* delivered . . .' (*The Correspondence of Jonathan Swift*, ed. H. Williams (Oxford, 1963-5), i. 174).

58. The Marlboroughs had four children living in 1710, all daughters, their only son having died in 1703. These were Henrietta, Anne, Elizabeth, and Mary. Sarah had four posts—groom of the stole, keeper of the privy purse, mistress of the robes, and ranger of Windsor Forest, none of which went to any of her daughters. Luttrell recorded on 20 Jan. 1711 that the 'dutchesse has resign'd her places, except that of ranger of Windsor forest, which is for life; the dutchesse of Somerset will succeed as groom of the stole, Mrs. Masham as privy purse, and the lady Hyde as lady of the robes' (Luttrell, vi. 680).

59. Thomas Erle (?1650–1720) was a high-ranking army officer, lieutenant-general in 1707 and commander-in-chief in England and Wales, and governor of Portsmouth in 1709. He was on very good terms with the Duke of Marlborough, safeguarding the Captain General's interests against the committee at the War Office which the Harley ministry set up in 1711 to take over the supervision of promotions in the army (I. F. Burton, 'The committee of Council at the War-Office', *Historical Journal*, 4 (1961), 78–84; Drax MSS.: Churchill College, Cambridge; Marlborough to Erle 16 Apr. 1711).

60. The letter is printed in *Priv. Corr.* i. 367–9: The Duke to the Duchess of Marlborough, 30 Aug. 1710 (NS).

61. At the time of Godolphin's dismissal 'lest the Court of Hanover should either upon their own observations, or the suggestions of the discontented Whiggs, take umbrage at the present and intended Alterations, her Majesty appointed Richard Earl Rivers to go immediately her Envoy Extraordinary to that Court, to remove all Jealousies' (Boyer, *Annals*, ix. 237).

62. There is little evidence to support Sarah's suspicions, that Harley was antipathetic to the House of Hanover. He was after all the chief architect of the Act of Settlement of 1701 which vested the succession in that House. And at the time of this entry there were rumours that Rivers had been 'sent by her majestie on some private message, some say, to offer the command of our army in Flanders to that prince [the Elector]' (Luttrell, vi. 616). The Marlboroughs apparently believed these rumours (Coxe, iii. 126, 128). The belief that he was prepared to offer to replace the Duke of Marlborough with the Elector of Hanover scarcely squares with the notion that Harley was prejudicing Anne against that family.

63. Among the addresses presented to Queen Anne in 1710 there were eleven from the clergy (see *A collection of the addresses which have been presented to the queen since the impeachment of the Reverend Dr. Henry Sacheverell* (1710)). Of these ten could be described as 'from the Countrey', but the one that caused the most controversy was from the bishop and clergy of London, presented on 22 August. Although this was scarcely 'from the Countrey' it 'was taken notice of', in that it had attracted country-wide attention for its attempt to reconcile the doctrine of passive obedience with support for the Revolution and the Hanoverian succession. It spoke of Anne's 'irresistible authority' and of how they had 'vigorously and successfully withstood' James II. Its inconsistencies were commented on in the *Observator*, 25 Aug. 1710.

64. The print *Queries* (p. 76 n. 54) generated a number of Tory replies, including *Counter Queries* and *Queries for Queries*. It is unlikely that either of these was the one which Hamilton gave to the Queen. Although a tract with the exact title he supplies here does

not appear to have survived, a Whig tract with the title *Queries number II* came out shortly after the presentation to the Queen of the address from the London clergy, and could conceivably be that referred to here.

65. *A letter concerning allegiance, written by the lord bishop of L . . . . n* was published on 12 Sept. (*Daily Courant*, 12 Sept. 1710). In fact two letters of Bishop Compton were published together, the one mentioned in the title, in which he had opposed the doctrine of non-resistance, and an extract from *The bishop of London's seventh letter at the conference with his clergy held in the year 1686*, first published in 1690. After the letters were printed thirty-five queries, which have been attributed to Benjamin Hoadly, in support of some Whig clergymen who had refused to sign the address.

66. *A Test offer'd to the consideration of the electors of Great Britain* accused the Tories of Jacobitism, and republished a blacklist drawn up in 1703 of those Tory M.P.s alleged to be opposed to the House of Hanover.

67. Henry Boyle (d. 1725) had been in office since 1701, as Chancellor of the Exchequer until 1708 and then as Secretary of State. He resigned on 20 Sept. (Boyer, *Annals*, ix. 241). He was an old acquaintance of Harley, who tried to persuade him to stay in office (HMC *Portland* ii. 220).

68. There were two tracts with this short title: *Now or Never: or, a project under God to secure the Church of England. in a congratulatory letter to the right honourable the earl of D . . . upon his late promotion*; and the same 'answer'd paragraph by paragraph. By a well-meaning Tory, who is willing to clear the Church of England from Jacobitism'. The first of these is rare—Professor Calhoun Winton opined that the copy of it at the Library Company of Philadelphia was unique (*The Augustan Milieu* (1970), p. 143 n. 1), but there is another copy at Yale. Presumably Hamilton showed Anne the second, which stresses the dangers of religious intolerance.

69. Samuel Clarke (1675–1729) D.D., rector of St. James's Westminster, published the *Scripture Doctrine of the Trinity* in 1712 and was accused of Arianism in 1714. He was a low-church Whig divine.

70. *A letter to the Examiner printed in the year 1710* laid down the policy to be pursued by the new Tory weekly. This was to paint the present state of the war abroad and to expose the ill practices of the Junto (it is reprinted in Boyer, *Annals*, ix, Appendix, 64–70).

71. *An Essay upon Publick Credit* attempted to demonstrate that the previous ministry had not enjoyed a monopoly of public credit and that the Harley ministry would be financially viable (see p. 75 n. 48).

72. Charles Davenant (1656–1714) was inspector-general of imports and exports from 1705 to 1714 and one of the leading economists of the age. Besides his tracts on economic subjects he also wrote political pamphlets: e.g. *Essays upon the balance of power* (1701) and the more readable *A true picture of a modern Whig* (1701). Cowper dealt with the tracts mentioned here as though they were by the same author in his own pamphlet *A letter to Isaac Bickerstaff Esq; occasion'd by the Letter to the Examiner* (reprinted in Boyer, *Annals*, ix, Appendix, 71–90). Although he did not name the writer he apparently thought it was

Davenant, since Hamilton almost certainly put this to the Queen after consulting with Cowper.

73. Apparently Anne was prepared to leave Hamilton and Cowper under the mistaken impression that the two tracts were by the same author, since if she really knew who had written them she could have told them that the *Letter to the Examiner* was by Henry St. John and the *Essay upon Publick Credit* was by Daniel Defoe.

74. Shortly after his trial Sacheverell left London to take up the living of Selattyn in Shropshire. His journey through the Midlands to the borders of North Wales soon turned into a triumphal procession (Holmes, *Trial*, pp. 242–8). Harley feared that Sacheverellite agitation threatened to produce a Tory landslide if parliament were to be dissolved, and Daniel Defoe, who had by now entered the service of the new ministry, in his *The Banb . . . y Apes* ridiculed Sacheverell's reception at Banbury. He made much of *Dr. Sacheverell's disappointment at Worcester* and finally disparaged the whole journey in *A New Map of the laborious and painful travels of our blessed high church apostle*. Anne's comment, therefore, probably reflects the attitude of her new Prime Minister to the effects of Sacheverell's tour.

75. Benjamin Hoadly (1676–1761), lecturer of St. Mildred's Poultry, London, from 1701 to 1711, was the leading low-church champion of the doctrine of resistance.

76. Peregrine Osborne (1658–1729) was the son of Sir Thomas Osborne (1631–1712) and succeeded to his father's titles as he moved up the peerage. Though he was summoned to parliament as Baron Osborne he was known as Earl of Danby from 1689, when his father was promoted from that honour to the Marquisate of Carmarthen, until 1694, when his father became Duke of Leeds and he adopted the title of Marquis of Carmarthen. In 1712 he succeeded his father as second Duke of Leeds. In Anne's reign all his recorded votes in the House of Lords were on the Tory side (Holmes, p. 429).

77. Although Anne dismissed the story coolly to Hamilton she had not been prepared to overlook it altogether. The Attorney-General and the Solicitor-General had been alerted to investigate 'several particulars . . . heard from the lady whom my lord Carmarthen marryed last, about a plot for imprisoning the Queen and settling the Pretender on the throne' (PRO/SP/34/13/31), and they had compiled a dossier on the incident (PRO/SP/34/13/31–33, 62). A letter from Bishop Burnet describes her as the lady 'who calls herself lady Carmarthen', while another identifies her as 'Mrs. Mary Morton with whom my Lord keeps company, and who as he has heard pretends to have been marryed to his Lp'.

78. William Cowper, first Earl Cowper (d. 1723) was made Lord Keeper of the Great Seal on 16 Oct. 1705, when he was still Sir William Cowper Bt., largely by the intercession of Godolphin and the Marlboroughs with the Queen. On the day of his appointment he wrote to the Duke of Marlborough 'I visibly owe [the honour] to the sole favour and goodness of my lord Treasurer, so I beg leave of your Grace at the same time to believe and confess with the utmost gratitude the power of your Grace's unseen hand in this my promotion . . .' (Blenheim MSS., AI: 26).

79. Hamilton seems to have got the date wrong here, for it was on 22 September that Cowper noted in his diary how he had tried to surrender the Great Seal to the Queen. 'She strongly oppos'd my doing it, giving it me again at least 5 times after I had laid it down,

& at last would not take it, but commanded me to hold it, adding "I beg it as a Favour of you, if I may use that Expression:" on which I took it again; but after some pause told her, "I could not carry it out of her Palace, unless she would promise me to accept to Morrow of it, if I brought it;" which I think she did, saying, she hoped I wod alter my Mind . . .' (Cowper, *Diary*, pp. 46–7).

80. Although Cowper noted in his diary that he had given the queen 'the Reasons of my Resolution to surrender, &c. (which, God willing, I will at leasure set down more at large)' (ibid., p. 46), no personal account by him has survived, so that this passage supplies information concerning Cowper's resignation not available elsewhere.

81. i.e. the Privy Council. On 21 Sept. Cowper noted 'The Council summon'd. Notice not at my House till about 1 o'clock, that I might have as little Notice as possible' (ibid., p. 45).

82. Sir Simon Harcourt (?1661–1727) had been Solicitor-General from 1702 to 1707, and Attorney-General from 1707 to 1708, when he resigned in sympathy with Robert Harley, who left the ministry at the same time. His loyalty to Harley was rewarded in 1710 when he became Attorney-General again on 19 Sept. and Lord Keeper on 14 Oct. (Luttrell, vi. 630, 643). In 1711 he was made Baron Harcourt.

83. There were four clerks of the Council at this time, William Blaithwaite, Edward Southwell, John Povey, and Christopher Musgrave; and three clerks extraordinary, James Vernon junior, Thomas Smith, and Abraham Stanion (J. Chamberlayne, *Magnae Britanniae Notitiae* (1708), p. 585; (1710), p. 515).

84. The proclamation dissolving parliament in 1710 referred to the Addresses in the following terms: 'And to the intent our good subjects may perceive the confidence we have in the assurances they have given us of their duty and affection, and how desirous we are to meet our people, and have their advice, by their representatives in parliament; we do hereby make known to our said subjects, that we do intend . . . to cause writs to be issued . . . for the calling a new parliament' (*Commons Journals*, xv. 398).

85. Faminianus Strada, *de Bello Belgico* (Rome, 1632–47).

86. Margaret of Austria, Duchess of Parma and Piacenza, illegitimate daughter of Charles V, Governess of the Spanish Netherlands 1545–68.

87. Anthony Perenott, Lord of Granville, a former Imperial ambassador, was made a cardinal in 1562 and was Margaret's principal adviser in the Netherlands from 1562 to 1564.

88. It is difficult to pinpoint the passage of Strada's *History* which Cowper had in mind, for as a Jesuit work it was written in favour of Margaret's measures and against those of the rebellious lords. However a letter sent by the lords to Philip II outlining their grievances against Granville was incorporated into the work, and this could be the source of Cowper's remark (*The History of the Low-Countrey Warres . . . written in Latin by Faminianus Strada; Englished by Sir Rob. Stapylton, Kt.* (1667), pp. 72–3).

89. 'Saturday Morn: 23 Septr. I waited on the Q. again; said I came now with an easier

heart than Yesterday, since her Majesty had pleas'd graciously to accept my Surrender, if I continued this Morning of the same Mind; which I did. Her Majesty answer'd, That she could use no more Arguments than she did Yesterday, but that she hop'd I would have chang'd my Mind: And thereupon I gave up the Seal, on my Knee; which the Q. accepted. Then I proceeded to advise her a little concerning my Succr. as, the day before, she had given me leave to do' (Cowper, *Diary*, p. 47).

90. Between the dissolution of parliament on 21 Sept. and the end of the month, besides a number of other changes at lower ministerial level and in the lord-lieutenancies, the following Cabinet changes were made: Sir Thomas Trevor, Robert Tracy, and John Scrope replaced Cowper as commissioners of the Great Seal until 14 Oct., when Harcourt became Lord Keeper; the Earl of Rochester succeeded Lord Somers as lord President; the Duke of Buckingham replaced the Duke of Devonshire as lord steward; Henry St. John obtained Henry Boyle's post of Secretary of State; and the Earl of Orford ceased to be first lord of the Admiralty. Lord Wharton resigned his post of lord-lieutenant of Ireland in September, but was not replaced by the Duke of Ormonde until 19 Oct. (Boyer, *Annals* ix. 241–4).

91. Samuel Bradford (1652–1731) obtained his D.D. from Cambridge University in 1705 and became a prebendary of Westminster in 1708. He had been a strong candidate the previous March for the bishopric of St. David's; Dyer actually reported his appointment on 14 Mar. 'upon the recommendation of his Grace of Canterbury' (BM Loan 29/310: cf. Luttrell, vi. 555), and on the same day White Kennett wrote 'Dr. Bradford I hope will be made easy in accepting the see of St. David's' (BM Lansdowne MSS., 1014, f. 110v). However, after the Sacheverell verdict, 20–1 Mar., the see remained unfilled for many months.

92. The person concerned has not been identified, but the reference may be to Lady Mary Cochran (see p. 103 n. 300).

93. There is no solid evidence to support Harley's statement that Cowper's resignation was concerted, but Speaker Onslow noted that Wharton had stiffened the Whigs, and especially Cowper, Halifax, and Somers, to resist Harley's overtures (Burnet, vi. 13, note), while Cowper went to the Privy Council meeting on the dissolution of parliament on 21 Sept. straight from a meeting at the Duke of Somerset's of Orford, Wharton, Somers, and the Dukes of Devonshire and Shrewsbury (Cowper, *Diary*, p. 45). It was perhaps at this meeting that Cowper's Whig colleagues pressed him to resign.

94. No pamphlet with this exact title appears to have survived, but among the election tracts which appeared after the dissolution was one published on 30 Sept. (*Observator*, 30 Sept.–4 Oct.) entitled *A letter to the good people of Great Britain* which is possibly that referred to here. It was a Whig letter, accusing the high-church Tories of being agents of France intent on destroying liberty and bringing back the Pretender.

95. Hamilton is presumably referring to the abortive bills to comprehend the Presbyterians in the Church of England. These had been introduced into parliament in 1680 and in 1689, while there were attempts to revive the measure as late as 1697 (H. G. Horwitz, 'Comprehension in the later seventeenth century; a postscript', *Church History*, 3 (1965), 1–7).

96. Rivers's initial reception at Hanover was cordial enough. As he wrote to Harley the

day after his arrival 'I cannot say enough of the kind reception I met with' (HMC *Portland* iv. 591). But the cordiality soon evaporated. On 13/24 Oct. he wrote 'I am left here alone the Court being all gone to a hunting seat' (ibid., p. 614). Lord Cowper noted in his diary that Rivers had been 'coldly reced' (Cowper, *Diary*, p. 49).

97. In May 1692 Anne had written to Sarah 'if you should ever do so cruel a thing as to leave me, from that moment I shall never enjoy one quiet hour. And should you do it without asking my consent (which if I ever give you, may I never see the face of heaven) I will shut myself up' (*Conduct*, pp. 75–6). The rumour that Sarah planned to publish her letters from the Queen got abroad. On 28 Nov. Henry St. John wrote to John Drummond 'Among other extravagancies [Sarah] now declares that she will print the queen's letters to her; letters writ whilst her Majesty had a good opinion of her, and the fondness for her, which her insolent behaviour since that time has absolutely eradicated' (Bolingbroke, *Correspondence*, i. 27). See Introduction, pp. xxxiv ff.

98. Presumably Hamilton was to try to prevent Sarah from seeing the Duke of Marlborough before he saw the Queen on his return to England. Marlborough left Holland on 23 Dec. and arrived in London on the 28th (Coxe, iii. 172).

99. The House of Commons discussed naval estimates on 5 and 6 Dec. (*Commons Journals*, xv. 416, 423; Luttrell, vi. 601). The debt on the naval accounts was estimated to be £5,131,539 at Michaelmas 1710, which occasioned some criticism of the previous ministry's financial management (*A letter to a friend concerning the publick debts, particularly that of the navy* (1711)). After hearing the second debate Arthur Mainwaring wrote to the Duchess of Marlborough 'their first vote was that the exceeding of the several sums granted by Parliament has been the chief occasion of the debts of the navy, and a violation of the rights of Parliament.' He goes on 'your friend Mr. Bathurst . . . reflected on the land service and concluded that the applying any part of the money given to the navy to the payment of the troops was a sad mismanagement etc. This has been done sometimes, tis true, but never without an absolute necessity, and the navy has always been repaid out of the pay of those troops . . . All the great successes of the war have been carried by those *exceedings* and *extraordinary payments* they have censured' (Blenheim MSS., E 27: 'Tuesday past six a clock').

100. ?George Churchill (1654–1710) Marlborough's Tory brother, who had been a naval commander in William's reign, and from 1702 to 1708 had been Prince George's principal adviser on the council of Admiralty, and had consequently borne the brunt of Whig attacks on the naval administration. He died in May 1710.

101. Three officers, Lieutenant-General Meredith, Major-General Maccartney, and Brigadier Honeywood, were cashiered about this time 'for drinking destruction to the present ministry, and dressing up a hat on a stick, and calling it Harley; then drinking a glass with one hand, and discharging a pistol with the other at the maukin, wishing it were Harley himself; and a hundred other such pretty tricks, as inflaming their soldiers and foreign ministers against the late changes at court' (Swift, *Journal*, p. 71).

102. The three officers were 'obliged to sell their commands at half value' (ibid.).

103. William Cadogan (1675–1726) was Marlborough's quartermaster and aide-de-camp from 1702 to 1711. 'Cadogan has had a little paring' Swift wrote to Stella on the 13th,

'his mother told me yesterday he had lost the place of envoy [to the Spanish Netherlands] but I hope they will go no further with him, for he was not at those mutinous meetings' (ibid.).

104. Algernon Seymour (1684–1750) was the eldest son of the Duke of Somerset, and hence took the title of Lord Hertford. In 1708 he went to Flanders as a volunteer, and returned in November with an express from the Duke of Marlborough about the relief of Brussels (Luttrell, vi. 297, 377–8). He was thus on good terms with the Duke, from whom doubtless he owed his promotion to the rank of lieutenant-general in 1709 (ibid., p. 503). What would mortify the Duchess, however, was his relation to the Duke of Somerset and the fact that he replaced as governor of Tynemouth Thomas Meredith, one of the Duke's favourites. It was an astute move, for Marlborough could hardly complain about Hertford's appointment since at the same time he had planned to give him the Duke of Northumberland's regiment if Northumberland succeeded Essex as constable of the Tower (Coxe, iii. 6–7).

105. Elizabeth Percy (1667–1722) married the Duke of Somerset in 1682. She had been a lady of the bedchamber since 1702, and succeeded Sarah as groom of the stole in January 1712.

106. 'on the 9th of December N.S. General Stanhope, with Eight English Battalions, and as many Squadrons, was attack'd in the Town of Brihuega, and forc'd to surrender Prisoners of War, after having defended that unfortify'd Place, as long as they had any Powder and Shot' (Boyer, *Annals*, ix. 118). The battle of Brihuega spelled the end of Allied hopes of placing Charles III on Philip V's throne by force of arms.

107. The text is Jas. 3: 17. The sermon was *An exhortation to purity and peace . . . preach'd in the parish-church of St. Mary le Bow by Samuel Bradford D.D. rector of the said church and chaplain in ordinary to her Majesty* (1710). In it Bradford asked 'Is it . . . a part of the Wisdom which is from above, when we are in danger from a common enemy without, thus by our intestine quarrels to lay ourselves open to him?' (p. 19).

108. Sir Nathan Wright (1654–1721) had been Cowper's predecessor as keeper of the Great Seal from 1700 to 1705.

109. Cf. Sarah's own accounts: 'I prevail'd with her Majesty to take the great seal from Sir Nathan Wright, a man despised by all parties, of no use to the crown, and whose weak and wretched conduct in the court of chancery had almost brought his very office into contempt' (*Conduct*, p. 147); 'For my Lord Cowper, I continually laboured with the Queen to make him keeper, to save the Duke of Marlborough and Lord Godolphin from an application so disagreeable to her; and at last, by a great deal of drudgery, I succeeded' (*Priv. Corr.* ii. 149–50).

110. John Somers (1651–1716) had been proposed to Anne as a Whig recruit to her ministry for many months before she made him lord President in October 1708. In April his Whig colleagues in the government had tried to persuade the Queen to take him into the Cabinet without giving him a ministerial post (Coxe, ii. 219). The Marlboroughs attributed the Queen's refusal to do even this to 'the power and inclinations of Mrs. Masham' (ibid., p. 214).

111. Edward Russell, Earl of Orford (1653–1727) succeeded the Earl of Pembroke as

lord Admiral in October 1709. (Cf. *Priv. Corr.* i. 224, 262, for Mainwaring's view that Sarah had been instrumental in procuring this appointment.) Allowing considerably for Mainwaring's flattery and exaggeration of Sarah's role, it does seem that Anne was minimizing it to Hamilton.

112. 'She used to entertain her confidents with telling them what a praying, godly idiot the queen was, and was wise enough to think they would keep such a secret for her: but Lady Fitzharding, who could not keep her secret in King William's time, was as little disposed to do it in queen Anne's' (Burnet, v. 454, Dartmouth's note).

113. Anne Churchill had married in 1700 Charles Spencer, who became the third Earl of Sunderland in 1702. She had been a lady of the bedchamber since Anne's accession.

114. Henrietta Churchill had also been a lady of the bedchamber since 1702. She had married Godolphin's son Francis, Lord Rialton in 1698, but was notoriously unfaithful to him. She was eventually to have an affair with, and a child by, Congreve. Even Sarah called her a 'fool' (Burnet, vi. 34, Dartmouth's note).

115. Mary Churchill had married Viscount Monthermer in 1704. He succeeded his father as Duke of Montagu in 1709.

116. John Montagu (? 1688–1749) was the second Duke of Montagu. In 1704 Sarah had obtained for him the post of Master of the Great Wardrobe for life (David Green, *Queen Anne*, p. 126; *Priv. Corr.* ii. 196).

117. For the text of Godolphin's memorandum to the Queen, sent via Hamilton, see Appendix D.

118. Marlborough's first interview with Anne after his return from abroad took place on 28 Dec., the day of his arrival. 'Upon the duke of Marlborough's coming home, I asked the queen, how she would have her servants live with him? She said, that would depend upon his behaviour to her, I told her, I was sure that would be all submission, since other means proved ineffectual; and asked her, if she could stand that? She said, from him she could. After he had been with her, she told me it was just as I said, only lower than it was possible to imagine' (Burnet, vi. 32, Dartmouth's note).

119. The Great Northern War between Sweden and Russia, which had broken out in 1700, took a new turn after the Swedish defeat at Pultava in 1709 when Charles XII fled to the Ottoman Empire and sought the aid of the Turks. In November 1710 the Grand Seigneur declared war on the Czar (Boyer, *Annals*, ix. 135), threatening the treaty of neutrality between the Grand Alliance and the Northern belligerents of March 1710 (ibid., Appendix 3). Troops were needed in Spain to replace those lost in the battles of Brihuega (9 Dec. N. S.) and Villaviciosa (10 Dec. N. S.). The French claimed that the allies had lost 14,000 men killed or taken prisoner during or after these engagements (Boyer, *Annals*, ix. 118, 129). 'Before the duke of Marlborough left the Hague, it had been resolved in a conference there, that all the troops ready in England and Ireland (about 7,000) should forthwith sail for Portugal' (Luttrell, vi. 671).

120. In an interview with Lord Dartmouth about this time the Duke 'complained of his wife, who, he said, acted strangely, but there was no help for that, and a man must bear with a good deal to be quiet at home' (Burnet, vi. 33, note).

121. John Campbell, second Duke of Argyle (1678–1743), who at the time of the battle of Oudenarde, where he had commanded the infantry, had been in the Duke's good graces (Coxe, ii. 260) was *persona non grata* with the Marlboroughs after his opposition to the Duke's request to be made Captain-General for life in 1709 (ibid., p. 492, note). At the time of the Sacheverell trial he voted the Doctor guilty, but opposed the votes imposing sentence upon him (ibid., iii. 26, note). He subsequently entered into all the intrigues of Harley, and in September 1710 replaced Marlborough's brother Charles as general of the English infantry in Flanders (Luttrell, vi. 633). He was elected a knight of the garter in March, but was not installed until 22 Dec. (ibid., pp. 560, 668).

122. Henry St. John (1678–1751) had an ambiguous relationship with Marlborough. Earlier in Anne's reign the Duke had been instrumental in obtaining the post of secretary at war for St. John in 1704 (Coxe, i. 152) and had even tried to keep him in the ministry in February 1708 when St. John chose instead to resign with Harley, though this intimacy was over by 1710. After St. John became Secretary of State in that year he regaled his correspondents with accounts of how the Duke's power had waned in England (Bolingbroke, *Correspondence*, i. 17, 38, 48–50). Even so he made endeavours to get back on good terms with the Duke himself (ibid. 71–2, 79–82, 115; I. F. Burton, 'The Committee of Council at the War-Office', *Historical Journal*, 4 (1961), 78–84).

123. George Granville (1667–1735) was a follower of Harley, who had obtained the post of secretary at war for him on 30 Sept. 1710 (Luttrell, vi. 635).

124. In his first interview with the Queen Marlborough 'pleaded fatigue, to shorten the visit' (Coxe, iii. 172).

125. This refers to Anne's last interview with Sarah, where she had told the Duchess repeatedly 'whatever you have to say, you may put it in writing', and 'you desired no answer, and shall have none' (*Conduct*, pp. 239, 241).

126. Mary of Modena (1658–1718) James II's Catholic queen.

127. 'And when upon the death of the PRINCE, one would have thought that her MAJESTY's real grief would have made her avoid every place and every object that might sensibly revive the remembrance of her loss, she chose for her place of retirement his closet, and for some weeks, spent many hours in it every day. I was amazed at this; and when I spoke to her of it, she seemed surprised, just like a person who on a sudden becomes sensible of her having done something she would not have done, had she duly considered. But the true reason of her Majesty's chusing this closet to sit in, was, that the back-stairs belonging to it came from Mrs. MASHAM's lodgings, who by that means could secretly bring to her whom she pleased' (*Conduct*, pp. 222–3).

128. According to Coxe the Duke of Marlborough, in order to discover the ministry's intentions with respect to Sarah, 'employed the intervention of Mr. Maynwaring, whose situation as one of the auditors of the imprest gave him frequent access to Harley. The result, however, contributed to increase his alarm, for the minister continually evaded every inquiry by the exclamation "that is the rock on which all will split, if care be not taken to avoid it"' (Coxe, iii. 174).

129. Cf. p. 82 n. 97.

130. See Appendix A, p. 108.

131. George Churchill, of whom Godolphin once wrote to Marlborough 'your brother does certainly contribute very much to keep up both in the Prince and in the Queen the natural, but very inconvenient averseness they have to the Whigs' (*Priv. Corr.* ii. 288). According to Coxe Sarah addressed 'a letter to the queen, full of bitter invectives, and declaring that all the brilliant services of the duke could not shield his brother against the clamours of the nation' (Coxe, ii. 356). 'The letter is lost' (David Green, *Queen Anne*, p. 173).

132. Ps. 15: 4 prophesies that among those who shall abide with God will be 'he that sweareth to his own hurt, and changeth not'. Ezek. 17: 18 predicts a judgement upon the king of Israel 'seeing he despised the oath by breaking the covenant, when, lo, he had given his hand'.

133. Marlborough was in the Tower from 5 May until October 1692 on suspicion of intriguing with the Jacobites.

134. Queen Mary's letter to her sister, requesting that she dispense with Sarah's services, was in fact written on 5 Feb. 1692, before Marlborough was confined in the Tower, but after his disgrace at Court (*Conduct*, pp. 43–7).

135. i.e. the one cited on p. 82 n. 97.

136. See Appendix A. The person is identified in the original contents list as the Bishop of Norwich (see Appendix C). Two days later, Hamilton read the opinion of the Bishop of Bangor to the Queen and, on the 22nd offered the views of White Kennett (ibid.).

137. See Appendix A.

138. See Appendix A. The key was the symbol of office of the groom of the stole.

139. The Duke of Shrewsbury. The House of Lords was involved from 4 Jan. to 10 Feb. in an inquiry into the war in Spain (Cobbett, *Parliamentary History*, vi. 935–97). They censured not only the Earl of Galway and General Stanhope, the English commanders in Spain, for the allied defeat at Almanza, but also the Cabinet ministers in office at the time for approving the strategy which led up to the battle, and for generally mismanaging the war. Shrewsbury opposed the previous ministry, while Cowper defended it, taking a leading part in the debates.

140. 'i.e. those employed in Harley's "scheme" of government' (Holmes, p. 401).

141. Swift referred to 'those Lords, who, by the Narrowness of their Fortunes, have depended on the Court' in a letter to Archbishop King, 8 Jan. 1712 (*The Correspondence of Jonathan Swift*, ed. H. Williams (Oxford, 1963–5), i. 284). There is an analysis of the 'poor Lords' and their parliamentary behaviour in Holmes, pp. 391–4.

142. On 9 Jan. Cowper, who had earlier been told 'that all the Scotch Lds of Parlt., except Annandale, were not able to live here without Money from the Q:', noted in his diary that a Whig attempt to avert censures on Galway and Stanhope by moving an adjournment of the committee had been defeated 'Yeas 45, Noes 59. Then main Qn

carried, without Division. Note, Not one Scotch Ld among the Yeas' (Cowper, *Diary*, pp. 51, 52). Cf. also Boyer, *Annals*, ix. 291.

143. By the 'wise and independent' Cowper presumably meant those 36 Whig peers who signed protests against the resolutions on the war in Spain on 12 Jan. (Cobbett, *Parliamentary History*, vi. 983, 985).

144. The title of Generallissimo had been conferred by Anne shortly after her accession upon her husband Prince George.

145. Adelaide Paleotti (d. 1726) married the Duke of Shrewsbury in Italy in 1706. Sarah detested her, writing to Lady Cowper on 25 Oct. 1710 complaining about her behaviour at Court 'entertaining everybody aloud, thrusting out her disagreeable breasts with such strange motions' (Panshanger MSS.).

146. John West, 15th Lord Delawarr (? 1663–1723) was groom of the stole and first gentleman of the bedchamber to Prince George from 1697 to 1708, and a civil-list pensioner from 1708 until he became treasurer of the chamber in 1713 (Holmes, p. 385).

147. Delawarr was a Court Tory, but very much more Court than Tory. He once left his proxy with a Whig lord—a very rare example of a peer leaving his proxy with a member of the opposite party—and on another occasion wrote 'I can truly say for myself that to support the Queen's interest in Parliament from the Revolution to this day has been always my study and my greatest ambition' (ibid., pp. 46, 386).

148. Two John Stewarts sat for Scottish constituencies at this time, both Whigs. John Stewart of Sorbie, member for Wigtownshire, 1707–27; John Stewart, member for Kirkcudbright 1708–15.

149. Mary Clavering (1685–1724) married Lord Cowper in 1706.

150. The Convocation of Canterbury met to do business on 24 Jan. On 29 Jan. Anne sent a letter to them with 'the heads of such matters as we think proper for the consideration of the said Convocation'. There followed nine items for their agenda, the first of which was 'The drawing up a representation of the present state of religion among us, with regard to the late excessive growth of infidelity, heresie and profaneness' (Boyer, *Annals*, ix. 328).

151. Anne was 'out of order and aguish' on 11 Mar. (Swift, *Journal*, p. 137). By 20 Mar. she was 'quite ride of her Ague. They keept it a secreet till the danger was past how many fitt she had had, so that when Dr. Ratclif heard her Phisitians had given her the Bark upon the first fit as he thought, he said the Elector of Hanover was to pay the Queen's Doctors' (*Wentworth Papers*, p. 188).

152. i.e. Sarah's daughter Anne, who was still a lady of the bedchamber.

153. Harley was raised to the peerage on 24 May 1711 as Baron Harley of Wigmore in the county of Hereford, Earl of Oxford and Earl of Mortimer (Boyer, *Annals*, ix. 381).

154. See Introduction, p. xxvi.

155. Richard Mead (1673–1754), who had been a member of the College of Physicians since 1708, was elected anatomy lecturer to the Barber-Surgeons on 16 Aug. 1711.

156. *Steel*: iron or steel filings administered internally; alternatively, the water in which iron or steel had been quenched when red-hot taken immediately or after being left for some days. Steel was supposed useful for spleen and dropsy.

157. Gilbert Burnet (1643–1715), Bishop of Salisbury since 1689, was interviewed by the Queen about this time to ascertain his views on the peace. This entry is presumably Anne's summary of the interview (for the Bishop's version see Burnet, vi. 77–8). The Dutch were being constrained because they could not afford to fight without England and yet were being offered less by the terms of peace than they had expected to receive.

158. In November 1711 the Marchioness of Gouvernet visited England with her son and daughter. The *Post Boy* of 22–4 of that month reported 'that the king of France had sent to the queen of Great Britain, by the marq. of Gournay, six complete suits, very magnificent, having caus'd the brocades to be made on purpose . . . his Majesty has order'd a sett of silver-gilt plate of a new invention for her'.

159. The tract has not been identified.

160. Earl Rivers went to Hanover as minister and plenipotentiary in October 1711, arriving there at the beginning of November. He waited on the Electoral Prince at Geure, and was back in London by 22 Nov. (*London Gazette* 25–7 Oct., 13–15 Nov.; *Protestant Post Boy* 22–4 Nov. 1711). While in Hanover the Elector gave him his opinion of the peace, which was far from complimentary (*Daily Courant*, 5 Dec. 1711).

161. Burnet's sermon does not appear to have been printed.

162. Cowper noted in his diary an interview with the Queen in December 1711 at which he was 'reced very kindly: she heard me above ½ an hour on the intended Peace; could not persuade me to promise to vote with Her Ministers' (Cowper, *Diary*, p. 53).

163. John Hervey (1665–1751) was created Baron Hervey of Ickworth in 1703 through Sarah's influence (*Conduct*, p. 127).

164. Anne began her speech at the opening of parliament on 7 Dec. 1711, 'I have called you together as soon as the publick affairs would permit, and I am glad that I can now tell you, that notwithstanding the Arts of those who delight in War, both Place and Time are appointed for Opening the Treaty of a General Peace' (Boyer, *Annals*, x. 282). 'The speech gave occasion to many reflections: *the arts of those who delighted in war* seemed to be levelled at the duke of Marlborough and the preliminaries concerted at the Hague' (Burnet, vi. 78; cf. p. 73 n. 31 above).

165. On 7 Dec. the opposition in the House of Lords managed by one vote to add a clause to the address of thanks for the Queen's speech. The clause, suggested by the Earl of Nottingham, was 'to represent to her Majesty . . . that no peace can be safe or honourable to Great Britain, or Europe, if Spain and the West-Indies are to be allotted to any branch of the House of Bourbon'. The Court lost the vote largely because of the absence of Scottish peers who had not then arrived in London. On 8 Dec., therefore, they tried

to redeem their loss, by moving that consideration of the clause should be put off until their arrival, but this was defeated by 22 votes (Boyer, *Annals*, x. 284–8).

166. 'Ld Carmarthen was absent yesterday, but today was there and gave occasion for more confusion and disorder than has been usual in that Honble House' (Bod. Ballard MSS. 21, f. 176. [W. Delaune] to Dr. Charlett, Saturday [8 Dec. 1711]).

167. William Carey, 8th Lord Hunsdon (1684–1765) defies party classification, being a peer 'who voted Dr. Sacheverell guilty side by side with the warmest Junto lords in March 1710, yet whose backing Harley never doubted from the very start of his ministry . . . He even supported the Schism bill in 1714 with the same aplomb with which he had condemned the arch-enemy of the schismatics in 1710' (Holmes, p. 385).

168. 'What he actually acquired was a bounty of £1000—this in addition to a bonus of £200 paid him by the Lord Treasurer at the end of the previous session of Parliament' (ibid., p. 515, note 8).

169. Cowper was minimizing the extent of Harley's parliamentary management in his attempts to reverse the hostile vote of the previous day. For example 'It was by many expected, That the Court Party would, the next Day, have the Majority, by means of the Proxies, which Eight Scotch Peers had sent to the Duke of Hamilton and the Earl of Marr' (Boyer, *Annals*, x. 288).

170. The ministerial riposte to the Earl of Nottingham's motion on the 7th was 'that in all probability few of the Members of the House were prepared to speak to it, but that it might be debated at a more convenient time'. The Whigs swept this objection aside, Lord Sunderland asking 'Is it possible that any members of this Illustrious House should be unprepared to debate an Affair which for these Ten Years past has been the principal subject matter of our consultations?' (Boyer, *Annals*, x. 284–5).

171. Harley's reply to Nottingham's motion was 'That according to the rules and orders of the House, this was not the proper time to debate such a motion'. It appears to have been Wharton who responded immediately by denying that 'there were any such orders' (ibid., p. 285).

172. Apparently Cowper was prepared to abandon the opposition to the peace preliminaries if the allies did not increase their proportion of the cost of the war effort. It is possible that he was persuaded to believe that the allied contribution was too low, and England's too high, by Swift's *Conduct of the Allies*.

173. It is possible that Hamilton has mistaken the date, since there was no significant debate in the Upper House on 14 Dec.

174. John, 1st Earl Poulet (1663–1743) had been first commissioner of the Treasury from August 1710 until 12 June 1711, when he was made lord steward (Boyer, *Annals*, x. 218). He was one of Harley's most valued followers.

175. Anne appears to be telling Hamilton about a recent debate in the Lords.

176. Anne's dislike of St. John at this time is well known. It was one of the reasons why

he was only promoted to a Viscountcy and not to an Earldom in July 1712, though he himself blamed Harley (*A letter to Sir William Windham* (1753), p. 31). Her adverse opinion of Harcourt, however, does not appear to have been previously noticed, though he had a reputation for being grasping, and had made a fortune at the bar.

177. John Holles (1662–1711) had been the moderate Whig whom Harley had brought into the ministry as lord privy seal in 1705. He had died on 15 July 1711 following a fall from his horse (HMC *Portland* v. 50).

178. Anne's answer to the address from the House of Lords included the expression 'I should be sorry anyone could think I would not do my utmost to Recover Spain and the West Indies from the House of Bourbon' (Boyer, *Annals*, x. 289).

179. Harley had seen Cowper on 18 Sept. 1710 to try to persuade him to stay in the ministry, and had told him that 'A Whig Game [was] intended at bottom' (Cowper, *Diary*, p. 43).

180. Presumably the terms offered to France at The Hague in 1709 and again, with only slight modifications, at Gertruydenberg in 1710. This is remarkable, since Cowper had previously thought that the Hague preliminaries were too severe on Louis XIV (ibid., p. 41).

181. On 28 Nov. Baron Bothmar had presented a memorial to St. John from the Elector of Hanover, complaining that 'In these [Preliminaries] there is neither any real security, nor any clear and distinct declaration'. It particularly urged that Philip V should not be allowed to keep Spain and the Indies (Boyer, *Annals*, x. 270–6). 'This memorial . . . a few days after it was presented, was made publick in a news-paper called the *Daily Courant* . . . many thousands of it were immediately sold off, and some printed on a large sheet to be preserv'd in frames' (ibid., p. 277).

182. Daniel Finch, 2nd Earl of Nottingham (1647–1730) had been Secretary of State from 1702 to 1704, but was left out of the ministerial reconstruction of 1710.

183. Hamilton's 'they' is puzzling, whether it refers to the ministers or the Whigs. In fact 'by the time Nottingham arrived in London late in November 1711, he was determined to oppose the peace "though no Man else would, if Spain and the Indies were to go up to the Duke of Anjou"' (H. Horwitz, *Revolution Politicks* (Cambridge, 1968), p. 229). He agreed to join the Whigs in opposing the preliminaries on condition that they would vote for an occasional conformity bill (ibid., p. 231).

184. Hamilton must mean Henry St. John, who was not created Viscount Bolingbroke until July 1712, since the previous Lord Bolingbroke, the last Earl, had died in 1711.

185. Nottingham himself charted the progress of the Bill and described the efforts of the ministry to frustrate his measure in a long letter to his wife of 26 Dec. 1711 (Northants RO, Hatton–Finch MSS., 281). The Harleyites tried to stop the Tories adding a penalty clause, but Nottingham forestalled them.

186. James Douglas, 4th Duke of Hamilton (1658–1712) was elevated to the British peerage as Baron Dutton and Duke of Brandon on 10 Sept. 1711. Constitutionally the

promotion was regarded as an infringement of the Act of Union which limited the representation of Scottish peers to sixteen (see Burnet, vi. 88). Politically the opposition was very concerned to prevent the government increasing the number of dependent Scottish lords in order to obtain an over-all majority (Geoffrey Holmes, 'The Hamilton Affair of 1711–1712: a crisis in Anglo-Scottish relations', *English Historical Review*, 77 (1962), 257–82). On 20 Dec. the opposition managed to carry by 57 votes to 52 the resolution 'that no Patent of Honour granted to any Peer of Great Britain who was a Peer of Scotland at the time of the Union can entitle such Peer to sit and vote in Parliament or to sit upon the Trial of Peers' (ibid., p. 267).

187. Relations between the Queen and some of her ministers were strained following the defeat of the government in the House of Lords on 7 Dec. Swift expressed their misgivings to Stella on 9 December: 'I was this morning with Mr. Secretary [St. John]; we are both of opinion that the Queen is false . . . I then went to my friend [Erasmus] Lewis [Dartmouth's under-secretary] . . . He talks of nothing but retiring to his estate in Wales. He gave me reasons to believe the whole matter is settled between the Queen and the Whigs' (Swift, *Journal*, p. 297).

188. The solution Harley persuaded the Queen to adopt in order to overcome their difficulties in the House of Lords astonished even some of his closest colleagues. 'I was never so much surprised' Lord Dartmouth later observed 'as when the queen drew a list of twelve lords out of her pocket, and ordered me to bring warrants for them; there not having been the least intimation before it was to be put in execution.' (Burnet, vi. 94–5, note.)

189. i.e. Marlborough.

190. i.e. if James II had created peers there would have been no Revolution in 1688.

191. Presumably Lord Cowper. When Cowper saw the Queen in December they had discussed the Hamilton patent as well as the peace, and 'in speaking on this subject [she] was pleas'd to say to me, "That the House of Lords was already full enough. I'll warrant you, I shall take Care not to make them more in hast" '. His next entry in his diary is without comment: 'Janry 2d. Twelve new Lds introduced, —3 by Writt, & 9 by Pat.' (Cowper, *Diary*, p. 53).

192. Anne told Dartmouth that 'she had made fewer lords than any of her predecessors' (Burnet, vi. 95).

193. Marlborough's opposition to the peace preliminaries was the final parting of the ways between him and the ministry. On 22 Dec. the commissioners of public accounts reported to the Commons an accusation that the Duke had profited corruptly from the supplying of bread to the army in Flanders (Boyer, *Annals*, x. 299). On 31 Dec. the Queen noted in Cabinet that '[she] thought fit to dismiss him from all his employments, that the matter might undergo an impartial investigation' (Coxe, iii. 280). On 1 Jan. she sent a letter to Marlborough with this message, which the Duke threw promptly into the fire (ibid.).

194. The *Post Boy* of 5–8 Jan. contained the following advertisement: 'yesterday morning a manuscript upon a whole sheet of paper was lost, wherein amongst other matters,

contain'd a particular account of the C... ss of S.... s poysoning 47 persons of quality... whoever brings them to Aby, at Jenny Man's, shall have a guinea reward'. This was an allusion to prince Eugene's mother, Olympia, countess of Soissons (1638–1708) who was banished from France in 1673 suspected of having poisoned her husband and of being involved in a plot to poison Louis XIV.

195. See p. 74 n. 32.

196. John Arbuthnot (1667–1735) was, thought Swift, 'the Queen's favourite physician' (Swift, *Journal*, p. 239). He was also a Tory writer, member of the Brothers and Scriblerus Clubs, and had just 'had the greatest share' in the compilation of a political ballad published on 4 Jan. (ibid., p. 311), though his most celebrated work, *Law is a bottomless pit*, which created the character of John Bull, did not appear until later in the year.

197. Among the disciplinary measures taken by the ministry in order to assert its authority in parliament was the dismissal of the Whig duke of Somerset from his post of Master of the Horse on 17 Jan. (Boyer, *Annals*, x. 315). Some wanted to go further and to remove the Duchess of Somerset from her posts of groom of the stole and first lady of the bedchamber. But though 'she had offer'd to resign . . . Her Majesty would not consent to part with so Trusty and Affectionate a Servant' (ibid.).

198. 'He [Somerset] was a man of vast pride, and having had a very low education, shewed it in a very indecent manner. His high title came to him by one man's misfortune, and his great estate by another's; (for he was born to neither, but elated with both to a ridiculousness.)' (Burnet, vi. 14–15, Dartmouth's note). For Cowper's efforts to prevail upon Somerset to allow his wife to remain in Anne's service see Holmes, p. 215.

199. 'The duchess of Somerset was the best bred, as well as the best born lady in England' (Burnet, vi. 34, Dartmouth's note). The obvious comparison is with the low-born Abigail.

200. 'She maintained her dignity at court, with great respect to the queen, and civility to all others' (ibid.).

201. Popular rumour was so certain that the Duchess of Somerset was on the verge of resigning on 25 Jan. that the Duchess of Hamilton, who was held to be the favourite to succeed her, was reported to have 'made her stays of late with loops for the gold key' (*Wentworth Papers*, p. 258).

202. On 25 Jan. the Lords were in committee on the constitutional issues raised by the resolutions on the Duke of Hamilton's patent making him Duke of Brandon (see p. 90 n. 186: Geoffrey Holmes, 'The Hamilton Affair of 1711–1712', 274).

203. Jonathan Swift wrote the *Windsor Prophecy* on 23 Dec. 1711. By the 24th it was in print, and designed to be published after Christmas Day. On the 26th he saw Abigail Masham who 'desired me not to let the Prophecy be published, for fear of angering the Queen about the Duchess of Somerset; so I writ to the printer to stop them. They have been printed and given about, but not sold' (Swift, *Journal*, pp. 304–5). But the printer did not get the letter, and enough copies circulated to give it wide publicity, with disastrous consequences to Swift's career (see Philip Roberts, 'Swift, Queen Anne, and *The Windsor Prophecy*', *Philological Quarterly*, 49 (1970), 254–8).

204. The following lines in the *Windsor Prophecy* relate to the Duchess of Somerset, called 'Carrots' because her hair was red:

> Their Conyngs mark[a] thou, for I have been told,
> They Assassine when young, and Poison when old.
> Root out these Carrots, O Thou whose Name
> Is backwards and forwards always the same[b];
> And keep close to Thee always that Name,
> Which backwards and forwards is allmost the same.[c]
> (Swift, *Poetical Works*, ed. Herbert Davis (Oxford, 1967), p. 97)

[a] The Duchess's second husband, Thomas Thynne, was murdered in 1682 by assassins hired by a rival suitor, Count Konigsmark.
[b] Anna. [c] Masham.

205. Jonathan Swift (1667–1745) entered Harley's service as a government propagandist in November 1710 when he wrote *Examiner* no. 13. He continued to write the *Examiner* until the following June. In November 1711 he published *The Conduct of the Allies* and *An Excellent New Song, being the intended speech of a famous orator against peace* [Nottingham] (Cf. *Priv. Corr.* ii. 138).

206. The deanery of Wells. William Graham, the dean, died on 4 Feb. 1712, and on the 5th Swift wrote to Harley to apply for the living (Swift, *Corr.* i. 288 and note: Roberts, loc. cit., p. 257).

207. The Act of Union of 1707 recognized the Presbyterian Church as the established church in Scotland, and made no provision for the toleration of other sects, much to the chagrin of high-church Tories in England who feared for the episcopalian ministers who used the Anglican liturgy north of the border. On 21 Jan. 1712 a bill was introduced into the Commons granting toleration to ministers who used the book of Common Prayer in Scotland. On 15 Feb. the bill, with amendments, passed the Lords (Boyer, *Annals*, x. 363). 'one clause put in it occasioned great complaints; the magistrates, who by the laws were obliged to execute the sentences of the judicatories of their kirk, were by this act to execute none of them' (Burnet, vi. 106). For Presbyterian objections that this exempted all but members of the established church from the jurisdiction of judicatories see *The Lockhart Papers* (1817), i. 379–80.

208. For the societies for the reformation of manners see D. W. R. Bahlman, *The Moral Revolution of 1688* (1957).

209. Perhaps his matrimonial problems. See Introduction, p. xxi.

210. On 6 June the Queen had communicated the general terms of peace to parliament in a speech (Boyer, *Annals*, xi. 111–17). The independent Whig Lord Hervey was not a particularly assiduous attender of debates.

211. 'June 1712. I waited on Q. at Kensington by appointment, procur'd me by Sr. D[avid] H[amilto]n: discoursed of the intended Peace . . . I endeavour'd to explain the Fallacy of the intended Renunciation's executing itself, &c.' (Cowper, *Diary*, p. 53). Cowper was objecting that Philip V's renunciation of his claim to the throne of France in the peace treaty could not be relied upon, and insisted that proper guarantees for the observation of the terms by France and Spain should be obtained.

212. In the Lords' debate on the Queen's speech Cowper had opposed Strafford's attack on peers who corresponded secretly with the allies to persuade them not to join in the peace treaty (see Cobbett, *Parliamentary History*, vi. 1146). He led demands for a clause to be added to the address requesting a guarantee that the terms would be honoured by France and Spain, but these were defeated by 81 votes to 36 (ibid. 1147), the heaviest Whig defeat in the House of Lords in the whole of Anne's reign.

213. In her speech Anne had told the Houses that 'The safety of our home trade will be better provided for by the demolition of Dunkirk' (ibid. 1143). The Whig lords protested on 10 June that this was not being carried out (ibid. 1150). Dunkirk had been a haven for French privateers who had considerably harassed English merchant shipping during the war (J. S. Bromley, 'The French privateering war', *Historical Essays 1600–1750 pres. to David Ogg*, ed. H. E. Bell and R. L. Ollard (1963)).

214. This presumably refers to the towns in the Netherlands which were to be garrisoned by the Dutch as a barrier between the United Provinces and France. A number of barrier towns were dropped in 1712 when the Tories renegotiated the treaty of 1709. According to Anne the Dutch had been guaranteed 'the entire Barrier, as demanded by the States in 1709 from France, except two or three places at most' (Cobbett, *Parliamentary History*, vi. 1143–4). The Whig lords, including Cowper, protested that this 'will render their Barrier wholly insufficient, and consequently very much weaken the security of Britain' (ibid. 1150).

215. In her speech Anne assured the Houses of 'the removal of that person out of the dominions of France, who has pretended to disturb this settlement' (ibid. 1142). The Pretender had to leave France and reside in Lorraine. Yet he did not go immediately, for despite rumours that he had withdrawn from Saint-Germain to Lorraine in June, he was still in Paris in August (Boyer, *Annals*, xi. 211–12, and see below, n. 218).

216. ?Robert Keith (1681–1757), or possibly George Keith (1639?–1716). *Vid. DNB.*

217. The *Daily Courant* of Saturday 6 Sept. 1712 published a report 'from the Amsterdam Gazette, dated Sept. 13. Paris, September 5. The Duke d'Aumont will speedily set out for London, with his Dutchess. The Chevalier de St. George will not bear that name any longer, but that of Duke of Gloucester.' The story was *not* reported in the *Post Boy* of 4–6 Sept.

218. Bolingbroke visited France from 2 to 21 Aug. (Boyer, *Annals*, xi. 203, 216). The *Flying Post* of 2–4 Sept. published the following report: 'The Harlem Courant of the 8th has the following news from Paris of the 2d . . . Last Friday as my lord Bolingbroke came to the Opera the king's box was appointed for him; but the Pretender coming thither he placed himself with his Governor, and the D. of Lauzune, in that Box; upon which the D. of Ossuna and my lord Bolingbroke were placed in a box over against him.' See H. T Dickinson, *Bolingbroke* (1970), p. 101.

219. i.e. gone out of the theatre.

220. See p. 93 n. 206.

221. Cowper is referring to the orders sent by Bolingbroke on 10 May to the Duke of Ormonde, Marlborough's successor as Captain-General, to prevent him from engaging

with the French (Bolingbroke, *Correspondence*, i. 500). The Whigs protested against the orders in a debate in the House of Lords on 28 May, but had been defeated 68 to 40. Twenty-five of the forty, including Cowper, had entered a formal protest in the Lords Journals (Boyer, *Annals*, xi. 102–6). As a result of the withdrawal of British troops the French under Marshal Villars were able to defeat the confederates at Denain in July and to take Douay (Burnet, vi. 135–6).

222. Cowper is here indulging in Whig fantasy. Very few of the Jacobites were in posts, nor were more than a tiny minority of those who held office under the Crown Jacobites. The Crown's ability to 'model' parliament to procure a Jacobite majority was minimal, as James II's own efforts to do so between 1685 and 1688 had proved. There was, however, to be an attempt to purge the army command of Hanoverian officers and to replace them with Jacobite sympathizers in 1714 (see Holmes, p. 28).

223. Cowper's reference to the Popish Plot of 1678 reveals its dominant place in Whig mythology. In fact Charles was originally informed as early as 13 Aug. 1678 that the Jesuits had laid plans to shoot, stab, and poison him (J. P. Kenyon, *The Popish Plot* (1972), p. 52).

224. After the prorogation of parliament a number of addresses were presented to the Queen from all parts of Britain to welcome the peace. The first, from the City of London, contained thanks to Anne for 'securing our trade in those parts where it hath been molested, by restoring it where it hath been lost, and by extending it to places to which it hath not, as yet, reached' (*London Gazette*, 14–17 June 1712). This set a pattern for a number of subsequent addresses, e.g. one from Windsor which asserted that the Queen 'has enlarged our trade, by extending it to coasts it never yet reach'd' (ibid., 7–11 October).

225. The South Sea Company was established in 1711, but was not allowed to trade with Spain's American possessions until 1713 (J. Carswell, *The South Sea Bubble* (1960), pp. 54–6). Those who bought goods in anticipation of an earlier concession from Spain had therefore to sell them at a loss.

226. The Portuguese trade had increased significantly since the signing of the Methuen Treaties in 1703, until the jeopardy in which it was to be allegedly placed by the Anglo-French commercial treaty became a major cause of the rejection of that measure by the Commons in 1713.

227. Pepys on 15 Oct. 1666 noted that 'This day the King begins to put on his Vest . . . being a long Cassocke close to the body, of black cloth and pinked with white silk under it, and a coat over it . . .'. The new fashion was doubly a war measure, being both economical and anti-French. Several courtiers, Thomas Killigrew presumably among them, wagered that the King would soon abandon it and the King was said to have accepted the bet at 100 to 1 (*The Diary of Samuel Pepys* ed. Robert Latham and William Matthews, vii (1972), 324, and n. 3). Marvell remarks on the King's habit of evading his promises in *The King's Vowes*, ll. 49–51.

228. i.e. Charles I.

229. The Whig newspaper, the *Flying Post*, in its issue for 6–9 Sept. 1712 carried an article 'on the Pretender's assuming the title of Duke of Gloucester' which argued that

'Every one knows this to be a Title belonging to the Royal Family of England, and that the last who enjoy'd it was that much lamented Prince her Majesty's own son', and concluded 'It is . . . very probable that he has chose this Title on purpose to affront the Electoral Prince of Hanover, whom her Majesty has lately created Duke of Cambridge'.

230. On 18 Sept. Swift informed Stella 'Yesterday we were alarmed with the Queen's being ill: she had an aguish and feverish fit; and you never saw such countenances as we all had, such dismal melancholy. Her physicians from town were sent for; but towards night she grew better, today she missed her fit and was up: we are not now in any fear; it will be at worse but an ague, and we hope even that will not return' (Swift, *Journal*, p. 383). On 9 Oct. he informed her that Anne was better (ibid., p. 386).

231. Richard Steele (1679–1729), the author, was official gazetteer from 1707 to 1710, and a commissioner of stamps from 1710 until 1713. In July Swift believed 'he will very soon lose his employment, for he has been mighty impertinent of late in his Spectators' (ibid., p. 376). By August, however, Steele had become much more accommodating to the ministry, writing to Harley on the 16th of his gratitude for Harley's generous treatment of him (HMC *Portland*, v. 211).

232. On 4 Nov. a would-be assassin sent a box to Harley containing two loaded pistols attached to the lid in such a way that they would go off when the box was opened. Swift, however, who was with him when it arrived, suspected a trap and dismantled the device (Boyer, *Annals*, xi. 294). When released in the press the story was widely disbelieved as a publicity stunt by the ministry, and Swift was much ridiculed, until he was goaded into publishing an account vindicating himself (Swift, *Journal*, pp. 393–4).

233. Hamilton informed Lord Cowper of this interview, for the latter noted in his Diary 'Novr 1712. Note. The Q: speaking to Sr Dd Hamn of the D. of Marlb. Intent to go abroad beyond Sea said, "He did wisely." By which I guess 'twas a kind of Composn between him & the Ministry, as well as for other Reasons' (Cowper, *Diary*, p. 54). Marlborough obtained a pass to go abroad on 30 October, and left England on 28 Nov. (Coxe, iii. 326–7).

234. Mrs. Judith Wilks testified to the birth of James Edward by signing a deposition at an extraordinary council meeting held on 22 Oct. 1688 (*Cal. S.P. Dom.* 1687–9, p. 327). It was part of Whig mythology that 'in this the midwife was the single witness; for none of the ladies had felt the child in the queen's belly' (Burnet, iv. 319), but there was other testimony (ibid., pp. 319–20, note).

235. See Introduction, pp. xxi–ii.

236. George Maccartney (? 1660–1730) was one of the officers cashiered in 1710 for taking pot-shots at an effigy of Harley (see p. 82 n. 101). He had been a second to Lord Mohun in the fatal duel fought with the Duke of Hamilton in Hyde Park on 15 Nov. According to one version of the duel Hamilton had killed Mohun, but was himself murdered by Maccartney, who made his way from England to Holland to escape justice. A notice for his apprehension was inserted in the *Gazette* on 2 and 6 Dec. (Boyer, *Annals*, xi. 301).

237. According to Dartmouth the Duchess of Somerset 'was by much the greatest favourite

when the queen died . . . Not long before the queen died, she told me she designed to leave some of her jewels to the queen of Sicily . . . and the rest to the duchess of Somerset, as the fittest person to wear them after her' (Burnet, vi. 34–5, note).

238. John Hamilton was the Duke of Hamilton's second in the fatal duel with Lord Mohun. He was brought to trial at the Old Bailey on 12 Dec. for the murder of Mohun, and found guilty of manslaughter (Boyer, *Annals*, xi. 310–11). The Tories took Hamilton's side, and the Whigs Maccartney's.

239. Anne in her speech opening parliament on 9 Apr. said 'The impious practice of duelling requires some speedy and effectual remedy', and a 'bill to abolish single combat; and to prevent the impious practice of duelling' was introduced in the Commons, but never became law (*Commons Journals*, xvii. 278, 281).

240. Swift observed on 25 Dec. 'the queen has the gout in her hand, and did not come to church today' (Swift, *Journal*, p. 405).

241. The Earl of Strafford went to The Hague in December 1712 to persuade the Dutch to accept the terms negotiated with France, and on 18 Dec. the States General expressed their willingness to do so (Boyer, *Annals*, xi. 313–29).

242. Isabella Danvers was one of the Queen's bedchamber women.

243. Mary, wife of John, 3rd Lord Ashburnham. She died 2 Jan. 1713. Swift, informing Stella of her death, wrote on 3 Jan. 'The poor creature was with child. She was my greatest favourite, and I am in excessive concern for her loss . . . She was naturally very healthy; I am afraid she has been thrown away for want of care' (Swift, *Journal*, pp. 409–10).

244. Mrs. Cotton has not been identified.

245. Mr. Beck remains unidentified. See p. 74 n. 32.

246. Jean Robethon (d. 1722), had been secretary to the Elector of Hanover since 1705.

247. Hugh Chamberlain (1664–1728) graduated M.D. at Cambridge in 1689 and became a Fellow of the College of Physicians in 1694. He was, like Hamilton, a celebrated *accoucheur* and a Whig. The incident Hamilton is describing remains obscure.

248. The Duc d'Aumont arrived in London on 2 Jan. 1713 as ambassador extraordinary from France. He achieved notoriety for distributing largesse in order to ingratiate himself with the people and the Queen. Many lampoons appeared against him (see W. Walker Wilkins, *Political Ballads of the Seventeenth and Eighteenth Centuries* (1860), ii. 136–40). Defoe ridiculed the notion that the Duke sold French wine duty free (*Review*, 22 Jan. 1713).

249. Probably a reference to a current libel on the Duchess of Shrewsbury, *The British Ambassadress' Speech*, in which the Duchess, who had accompanied her husband to Paris, is depicted as assuring Louis XIV that the ministry in England was fast implementing the French king's designs (there is a copy in the *Harleian Miscellany* (1809), iii. 325–7).

250. The *Flying Post* for 13–15 Jan. contained a story about a Protestant peer who had set aside his Catholic heirs and entailed his estate on a co-religionist by Act of Parliament. Having fallen out with the Protestant heir he was considering changing his mind and was presently being persuaded 'by an Act of Parliament to put it into his hands to leave his Estate by will to whom he pleases'. Defoe complained to Oxford that it had been received in Lincolnshire as evidence 'of a design in the next Parliament to settle the succession so as the queen shall leave it by will to whom she pleases' (HMC *Portland* v. 264, 267).

251. Hamilton is presumably referring to Whig allegations that the Tories had spent £13,000,000 of revenue which were unaccounted for, doubtless a riposte to Tory charges that there was £35,000,000 unaccounted for when Godolphin left the Treasury (*Commons Journals*, xvi. 611–13). The expression 'in time of peace' indicates a time before Anne's reign, and the implication that Nottingham was involved suggests the years 1679–84 when he was at the Admiralty Board (H. Horwitz, *Revolution Politicks* (Cambridge, 1968), pp. 20–38), and when the Earl of Rochester was first lord of the Treasury (see e.g. *The True Patriot Vindicated, or a justification of the late earl of Rochester* (1711)).

252. The tract has not been found, but its purport can be guessed from the story of Asa in 2 Chr. 16. Asa was condemned by a prophet because he had relied on the king of Syria and not on the Lord. 'And Asa in the thirty and ninth year of his reign was diseased in his feet, until his disease was exceeding great; yet in his disease he sought not to the Lord, but to the physicians.' Shortly after, he died. The disease was generally supposed to have been the gout.

253. *The new preface and additional chapter to the third edition of the Pastoral Care.* Burnet wrote the new preface to his *Discourse on Pastoral Care*, first published in 1692, on 15 Nov. 1712. In it he complained that 'the much greater part of those who come to be ordained are ignorant to a degree not to be apprehended by those who are not obliged to know it . . . They cry and think it a sad disgrace to be denied Orders, tho' the ignorance of some is such, that in a well regulated state of things, they wou'd appear not knowing enough to be admitted to the Holy Sacrament'.

254. Sir John Shadwell (1671–1747) was made physician extraordinary to the Queen in 1709 and physician-in-ordinary in 1712. Anne was ill at this time. On 4 Feb. Bolingbroke wrote to Shrewsbury 'the weakness remaining in the queen's feet after the pretty severe fit of the gout has been the principal motive for proroguing the parliament to the 17th instant' (Bolingbroke, *Correspondence*, ii. 233). The Duke and Duchess of Shrewsbury were then in France, the Duke having been made ambassador extraordinary for the final stages of the peace negotiations.

255. John Hamilton inserted a letter in the *Post Boy* of 7–10 Feb. 1713 denying that he had said that Maccartney had not killed the Duke of Hamilton, and insisting on the contrary that he 'saw Mr. Mackartney stabb his Grace'.

256. Edward Harley (1664–1735), Robert's brother, was one of the Auditors of the Imprest. Anne pressed Louis XIV to release Protestants from the French galleys, and in June the Duc d'Aumont gave Bolingbroke a list of 186 who had been released at the Queen's request, and who had left France, beside fifty others who remained (Prussian State Archives: Friedrich Bonet to Frederick I, 9/20 June 1713).

257. Sir Richard Vivian was knight of the shire for Cornwall and a Country Tory (Holmes, p. 117).

258. The abbot of Polignac was one of the French negotiators at Utrecht. 'The Night between the 10th and 11th of February [he] set out for the Court of *France*, on pretence of his being lately nam'd Cardinal by the Pope, at the recommendation as was, at this time and long before, reported of the person who *pretends to disturb the Protestant Succession in the House of* Hanover.' (Boyer, *Annals*, xi. 343.)

259. ? Richard Noble (1684–1713), an attorney who killed his mistress's husband and was executed for the crime on 28 Mar. 1713 (Swift, *Journal*, p. 449).

260. Thomas Trevor (1658–1730), chief justice of the common pleas since 1701, had been created Baron Trevor of Bromham as one of the dozen peers of 1712. He had declined the Great Seal in 1705 (Holmes, p. 204). According to lord Cowper he 'went violently into all the measures of that ministry, and was much trusted by them; and when they divided a little before the Queen's death, he sided with Lord Bolingbroke, and for so doing, 'tis credibly said, was to have been made Lord President' (Lord Cowper's *History of Parties presented to George I*, printed in Lord Campbell, *Lives of the Lord Chancellors* (1846), iv. 349–50).

261. Henry Grey (? 1664–1740) succeeded his grandfather as 9th Earl of Kent, and was elevated to the title of 1st Duke in 1710 as compensation for being deprived of the post of lord chamberlain by the Duke of Shrewsbury (see p. 73 n. 23). He was one of a number of Court Whig peers whom the ministers were courting at this time in an endeavour to maintain their majority in the Lords.

262. Lionel Sackville (1688–1765), 10th Earl of Dorset, was a Court Whig who occupied the post of lord warden of the Cinque Ports from 1708 to June 1713, when he was dismissed after having 'opposed the court in everything' (Holmes, p. 389).

263. 'Mrs. Harley' probably refers to Sarah, wife of Edward 'Auditor' Harley since 1695.

264. For the significance of Jewish investment in Bank and East India Company stock in Anne's reign, see P. G. M. Dickson, *The Financial Revolution* (1967), pp. 262–5.

265. The *Examiner* for 6–9 Mar. 1713 was devoted to countering the Whigs' 'Grand Epidemical Lye . . . that the Tories in Power are about to bring in Popery, a suggestion so monstrous and absurd, that one would think it were a little unreasonable to oblige us to apply any thing in the way of cure to a wretch so far gone, so irreparably lost in the deepest corruption of common sense, as to be capable of believing it'.

266. i.e. at the opening of parliament on 9 Apr., when Anne was to announce that treaties of peace between France and England, the United Provinces, Portugal, Prussia, and Savoy, had been signed at Utrecht on 31 Mar./11 Apr.

267. In her speech Anne said 'What I have done for securing the Protestant Succession, and the perfect friendship there is between me and the House of Hanover, may convince such who wish well to both, and desire the quiet and safety of their country, how vain all attempts are to divide us, and those who would make a merit by separating our interests,

will never attain their ill ends'. She also recommended to their care 'those brave men, who have served well by sea or land this war, and cannot be employed in time of Peace' (Cobbett, *Parliamentary History*, vi. 1172–3).

268. The House of Commons voted a unanimous address of thanks for the speech, but in the House of Lords some peers made objections to the Queen's reference to a general peace 'since the emperor, the elector of Hanover, and other princes and states of the empire, were not yet come into it'. A proposal to include in the address a clause asking the Queen to lay before the House the treaties of peace and commerce was defeated by 74 votes to 43 (ibid., p. 1174).

269. Charles VI, Holy Roman Emperor since the death of his brother in 1711, refused to come into the treaty of Utrecht, regarding it as a betrayal of the aims of the Grand Alliance. Although he was given until 1 June to declare his acceptance of its terms he refused, and did not make peace with Louis XIV until February/March 1714 when he signed the treaty of Radstadt.

270. Margaret, dowager Duchess of Newcastle (1661–1716) was the widow of John Holles, Duke of Newcastle, who had died in 1711.

271. Henrietta Cavendish (1693–1755), the Newcastle heiress, was the most desirable match in Europe, since her father had died an extremely wealthy man. Some estimated her income at £10,000 a year. She eventually married Harley's son Edward in August 1713.

272. Algernon Seymour (1684–1750), Earl of Hertford, married Frances Thynne in 1713.

273. See Roberts, loc. cit., p. 257.

274. James Edward's Protestation against the negotiations at Utrecht, addressed from Saint-Germain on 25 Apr. 1712, will be found, in Latin and French, in Lamberty, *Mémoires pour servir à l'Histoire du xviiie siècle* (The Hague, 1730), viii. 170–3.

275. See Roberts loc. cit., p. 268.

276. As part of the settlement at Utrecht the British government had negotiated a treaty of commerce with France. Unlike the peace treaty itself, which could be ratified without reference to parliament by virtue of the royal prerogative of declaring peace and war, this required parliamentary approval, since the eighth and ninth clauses removed tariff barriers previously put up against trade with France by statute.

277. Arthur Moore (? 1666–1730) had been a commissioner of trade and plantations since 1710. According to Burnet, when the treaty of commerce was put before the board for their opinion Moore 'moved that they might first read it every one apart, and then debate it; and he desired the first perusal: so he took it away, and never brought it back to them, but gave it to the lord Bolingbroke, who carried it to Paris, and there it was settled' (Burnet, vi. 163).

278. William Pierrepont, Earl of Kingston, only son of Evelyn, Marquis of Dorchester, died 1 July 1713.

279. Charles Trimmell (1663–1723), became Bishop of Norwich in 1708. He was the Earl of Sunderland's tutor.

280. On 14 May 1713 the House of Commons resolved 'That a Bill be brought in, to make effectual the eighth and ninth Articles of the Treaty of commerce and navigation between Great-Britain and France' (Cobbett, *Parliamentary History*, vi. 1213). France excepted from the reciprocal removal of tariffs, *inter alia* salted fish and the product of whales (Boyer, *Annals*, xi, Appendix, p. 188). Vivian was presumably interested, as knight of the shire for Cornwall, in the fate of the Devon and Cornish fishing industry.

281. Scottish dissatisfaction with the Union came to a head with the proposal to lay a duty of malt uniformly throughout Great Britain, which they claimed was an infringement of a clause in the Act of Union stating that there should be no duty on malt in Scotland during the war. Though peace was signed with France Britain was still technically at war with Spain. On 1 June the Scots peers joined with the Whigs in the Lords to propose a bill to dissolve the Union. The motion was lost by 71 votes to 67 (Cobbett, *Parliamentary History*, vi. 1215–19).

282. James Ogilvy (1664–1730), 1st Earl of Seafield, had succeeded as Earl of Findlater in 1711. He opened the debate on 1 June, summing up Scottish grievances under four heads, and moving that leave be given to bring in a bill to dissolve the Union (Cobbett, *Parliamentary History*, vi. 1216).

283. John Erskine (1675–1732), 6th Earl of Mar, seconded Seafield's motion on the 1st (ibid.).

284. On Monday 8 June the tension over the Malt tax reached its peak in the House of Lords when 'after a long debate which lasted 5 hours & much speeching on behalf of the poor Scotch the Bill was passed—Pros 64 Contras 56—the Whiggs & Scotch to a man joyned against it' (Berks. RO, Trumbull Additional MSS., 136/1: Ralph Bridges to Sir William Trumbull, 9 June 1713).

285. Sir David Dalrymple (d. 1721) was member for Haddington from 1708 until his death. He had been Lord Advocate until dismissed in 1711 for associating with the Whigs (Holmes, p. 243 and note 90).

286. The House of Commons debated the bill brought in to enact the eighth and ninth articles of the treaty of commerce with France on 18 June, when it was defeated by 194 votes to 185. Dalrymple voted against it (*A letter from a member of the House of Commons to his friend in the country relating to the bill of commerce* (1713)).

287. Possibly Julius Caesar, a physician who lived in Rochester. On Hamilton's visit to Rochester, see p. 22.

288. The Prussian chaplain has not been identified. He was presumably attached to Friedrich Bonet, the Prussian Resident in London.

289. The thanksgiving service for the peace, held in St. Paul's, was postponed from 16 June to 7 July because of Anne's illness. Even then she felt too ill to go, and attended service at St. James's instead (HMC *Bath* i. 235).

290. Thomas (b. 1695). See Introduction, pp. xx, xxiii.

291. 'Whereas Tipping's liquor, which is good against the stone and cholick, gout, etc hath had such great success in the cure of the aforesaid distempers, that it hath gotten it a name in the world; several persons . . . have made a spurious liquor, and father'd it by the name of Tipping. Near 20 of these counterfeits have risen and fell within these few years; and now one again, which is sprung from the same stock, has endeavour'd to carry on the cheat . . . My liquor is sold by Mr James in Three-King-Court in Lombard Street, and the widow Wakefield at the corner of Friday Street in Watling street' (advertisement in *Post Boy*, 1–3 Jan. 1712).

292. Mary Foyston was 'necessary woman to the Queen preferred to that employment by My Lady Masham' (Swift, 'An Enquiry into the Behaviour of the Queen's Last Ministry', *Political Tracts 1713–1719*, ed. H. Davis and I. Ehrenpreis (Oxford, 1953), p. 172 n.).

293. Of Anne's speech at the close of the parliamentary session on 16 July Burnet wrote 'few speeches from the throne have in my time been more severely reflected on than this was . . . The sharpness with which she expressed herself was singular, and not very well suited to her dignity or her sex . . . It was also observed that there was not, in all her speech, one word of the pretender, or of the protestant succession' (Burnet, vi. 178–9).

294. 'Crazy formerly meant cracked in the sense of being frail or indisposed' (David Green, *Queen Anne*, p. 289, note). Oxford was under considerable strain at this time on account of the struggle for power between himself and Bolingbroke which, up to the signing of the peace of Utrecht, and the subsequent proceedings in parliament, had been subordinated to the exigencies of policy. But 'by the end of the session . . . Bolingbroke had come to the conclusion that now was the time to make his bid for glory' (Geoffrey Holmes, 'Harley, St. John and the death of the Tory party', *Britain after the Glorious Revolution* (1969), p. 225).

295. Richard Hampden (1674–1728), Whig member for Wendover 1701–8, Bucks. 1708 to 1710, and Berwick in 1711. The Queen spoke angrily of an interview with him in Aug. 1710 (Holmes, p. 196; *Wentworth Papers*, p. 138) and when he stood in Bucks. in 1713, the *Examiner* of 20–4 July described him as 'a candidate . . . who lately went to Court under pretence of visiting the sick, and yet upon finding the person he went to in perfect health, discover'd such marks of regret and disappointment as entirely set aside the whole merit of a charitable disposition'.

296. Mrs. Smith has not been identified.

297. The *Flying Post*, 13–15 Oct. 1713, mentioned 'a late scandalous and surreptitious petition handed about gratis in the open streets for preserving the harbour of Dunkirk'.

298. *A short history of the parliament*, attributed to Robert Walpole, attacked the Tory majority in the 1710–13 parliament, alleging that they 'have sacrific'd their country to the power of France, which can end in nothing but bringing in the Pretender, Popery and Slavery' (p. 36). Thousands were printed and dispersed throughout Britain, while on 18 Sept. John Drummond wrote to inform Harley that 'the scandalous pamphlet called "The History of the late Parliament" is translated and printed at the Hague in Dutch and French' (HMC *Portland* v. 338).

299. The death of Emperor Joseph in April 1711 led to the election of his brother Charles, Habsburg candidate for the throne of Spain, as Holy Roman Emperor, in October. This unexpected development altered the balance of power in Europe, for if Charles got possession of Spain it would have meant the creation of an empire as large as that of Charles V.

300. The original contents list (Appendix C) identifies this person as Lady Mary Cochran, the eldest daughter of Alexander, Earl of Kincarden. She presented a memorial for arrears of pension in 1709, claiming £9,000. The claim dragged on and she received £100 from the Civil List on 13 Aug. 1713, £100 as royal bounty to carry her to Scotland on 14 Aug. 1713, and a further £100 on 9 Sept. 1713 (*Cal. Treas. Papers*, cxix. 7; *Cal. Treas. Books*, xxviii, pt. 2, 223–4; xxvii, pt. 2, 45, 321, 344).

301. In July and August the struggle at Court produced a major ministerial reshuffle, which 'ended in rout for Oxford's opponents' (G. Holmes, 'Harley St. John and the death of the Tory Party', p. 225). The Bishop of Bristol became Bishop of London and was replaced as lord privy seal by Lord Dartmouth. William Bromley succeeded Dartmouth as Secretary of State. William Benson was made Lord Bingley and sent as ambassador to Spain, Sir William Windham replaced him as chancellor of the exchequer, and Francis Gwyn took Windham's former post as secretary at war.

302. Parliament was dissolved on 8 Aug. and a General Election immediately ensued.

303. See p. 101 n. 287.

304. Elizabeth Harley, Oxford's daughter, married in December 1712 the Marquis of Carmarthen, grandson of the Duke of Leeds, who died in July 1712, and son of Peregrine, the Marquis of Carmarthen mentioned above, p. 79 n. 76, who succeeded his father as Duke of Leeds. Elizabeth died in childbirth on 18 Nov. 1713, to her father's great sorrow.

305. Mrs. Donnellen has not been identified.

306. Anne, who had been 'very well' on 3 Dec., was 'extremely ill' on the 24th (HMC *Portland* v. 369, 374). This was her most critical illness before her death, and for a while the Tories were 'out of their wits' (Swift, 'An Enquiry into the Behaviour of the Queen's last Ministry', p. 154).

307. See p. 88 n. 156.

308. See p. 102 n. 294.

309. On 5 Apr. the Lords had debated the succession, urging the Queen to issue a proclamation 'with a suitable reward for taking the Pretender, dead or alive, if he comes to Great Britain or Ireland . . . and a question was put whether the succession in the House of Hanover was in danger from her Majesty's administration. It was carried in the negative by fourteen' (HMC *Portland* v. 410). Presumably the idea was mooted that the succession could be secured by inviting over a member of the House of Hanover (see next note).

310. On 10 Apr. 'most of the Whig lords held a consultation at the lord Halifax's, to which

baron Schutz, envoy from the elector of Hanover was admitted. It was resolved . . . that the envoy should take the first opportunity to demand a writ for the Electoral Prince to sit in the House of Peers, as duke of Cambridge' (Cobbett, *Parliamentary History*, vi. 1341). On 12 Apr. Schutz saw the Lord Chancellor, who informed Harley: 'He told me he was commanded by the Princess Sophia . . . to demand of me a writ of summons to Parliament for the Duke of Cambridge' (HMC *Portland* v. 419). That night Harcourt saw the Queen and at a cabinet meeting it was agreed to grant the request (Cobbett, vi. 1342; HMC *Portland* v. 416–17). Harley reported 'I never saw her Majesty so much moved in my life' (HMC *Portland* v. 418). Cowper told Harley that had Schutz consulted him he would have tried to stop him (ibid. 440).

311. Steingens, the Palatine Resident 'who entertained relations both with lord Oxford and the Hanover Court' (W. Michael, *The Beginnings of the Hanoverian Dynasty* (1936), p. 35).

312. Matthias John, Baron Schulenberg (1661–1747) was brother to the Countess Ehrengard Melusina von der Schulenberg, a maid of honour to Princess Sophia and mistress of the elector of Hanover. A prominent Prussian soldier, he was a committed supporter of the Hanoverian succession.

313. 'The Queen you knowe was feaverish for two days, wch made her hasten from Kensington lying there but one night. She is now perfectly recovered' (Alnwick MSS. 22. i, f. 79: Lord Weymouth to Mrs. Thynne, 13 May 1714).

314. Steingens. See n. 311.

315. ? Schulenberg. See n. 312.

316. Plimpton remains unidentified.

317. Baron Schutz was ordered to return to Hanover as *persona non grata* after the storm he had created by applying for the duke of Cambridge's writ of summons to the House of Lords. When he returned to Hanover he was refused admission to the Court (HMC *Portland* v. 443, 447).

318. Thomas Harley, Robert's cousin, was sent to Hanover in Apr. 1714 to acquaint that Court with the English Ministry's account of the Cambridge writ affair, and returned to England in May (ibid., pp. 427, 437).

319. Edward Hyde (1661–1723), 3rd Earl of Clarendon, was sent as envoy to Hanover in June (ibid., p. 454).

320. George St. John (*c.* 1693–1716), Bolingbroke's half-brother, went as ambassador extraordinary and plenipotentiary to the Italian States, and as envoy extraordinary to Savoy, in July (D. B. Horn, *British Diplomatic Representatives 1689–1789* (Camden 3rd ser., 1932), xlvi. 72, 122).

321. Sophia died suddenly on 29 May in Hanover, at the age of eighty-four. An eyewitness thought that her sudden illness had been brought on by the correspondence from England about the Duke of Cambridge's writ. 'In the midst of this concern those letters

arrived, and those I verily believe have broke her heart, and brought her with sorrow to the grave' (Coxe, iii. 361). Had she lived three months longer she would have succeeded Anne as Queen Sophia under the terms of the Act of Settlement of 1701.

322. Chip in broth, pottage, porridge—'a thing or matter of no importance' (Eric Partridge, *A Dictionary of Slang* (1916)).

323. Isobell Hamilton (see Introduction, p. xix).

324. On 15 June Cowper was among the minority peers who protested against the schism bill to deprive dissenters of their separate schools. Amendments inserted by the Lords on 7 June exempted 'any person, who should instruct youth in reading, writing, arithmetic, or any part of mathematical learning, that relates to navigation, or any mechanical art only' (Cobbett, *Parliamentary History*, vi. 1355). These clauses nullified sections of the Act of Uniformity of 1662 which had forbidden any school to be set up without licence from a bishop.

325. There were rumours at this time that the Duke of Marlborough was to return to England. Bolingbroke took it for granted that he was returning in July, and that Harley was intriguing with him (Bolingbroke, *Correspondence*, ii. 670).

326. See p. 88 n. 156.

327. See p. 103 n. 300.

328. The Lords were hot on the scent of some dubious transactions between Arthur Moore and the Spanish government in the negotiations leading to the treaty of commerce with Spain. The secretary to the board of trade and plantations disclosed in the House 'that Mr. Moore had shewn him a letter in French from monsieur Orry, directed to don Arturio Moro, importing in substance, "That he must not expect the 2,000 louis d'ors per annum, that had been promised him, unless he got the three explanatory Articles ratified"' (Cobbett, *Parliamentary History*, vi. 1362).

329. Anne was anxious to end the session in order to stop the Whig inquiry into the negotiations over the Spanish treaty of commerce, but could not until a lottery bill was ready for the royal assent. When it was finally passed on 9 July she prorogued parliament until 10 Aug. (ibid. 1363–4). 'It was the general opinion that if the parliament had sat one day longer Mr. Moore would have been censured by the Lords and ordered to be prosecuted' (Boyer, *Political State*, viii. 17). Bolingbroke was even more anxious than the Queen to end the session and protect his creature Moore.

330. On 8 July the Lords had examined the Secretary and first clerk of the Treasury about the Assiento contract, whereby the South Sea Company was to be allowed to ship slaves to Spanish colonies. 'They confessed, that they were only nominal assignees for the quarter part of the Assiento contract reserved for the queen, and that some persons to them unknown (but who were strongly suspected to be the lord Bolingbroke, the lady Masham, and Mr. Arthur Moore) were to have the benefit of it.' Led by Cowper and Wharton the Whigs moved for an address to request the Queen to give her share to the South Sea Company. Next day Anne replied 'That she always had a great consideration for the advice of the House: and, as to the particulars desired, she would dispose of them, as she should judge best for the service' (Cobbett, *Parliamentary History*, vi. 1362–3).

331. Arthur Annesley (d. 1737), 5th Earl of Anglesey, was a high-church Tory who had been made joint vice-treasurer of Ireland in 1710. Since then, however, his voting behaviour had been very whimsical, and in the session of 1714 he 'steered a wildly erratic personal course . . . in a manner which suggests that his ambition for the viceroyalty of Ireland was more important to him than any of the causes he was ostensibly, and often eloquently, espousing' (Holmes, p. 279). He had moved the final form of address to the Queen on 8 July (Cobbett, *Parliamentay History*, vi. 1363).

332. Thomas, Earl of Wharton (1648–1715), was the leader of the Whig opposition in the House of Lords from 1710 to 1714. In the final debate of Anne's reign he threatened that the inquiry into the negotiations for the Assiento would be the first business to be raised in the House when it met again.

333. See textual note x p. 63. Thomas Coke (1674–1727) was vice-chamberlain of the household from 1706 to his death.

334. Cowper's children. He had one son by his first wife, and two by his second, William, b. 1709, and Spencer. He also had two daughters by his second wife.

335. Marlborough had resolved to return to England as soon as parliament was prorogued, and by 19 July was at Ostend awaiting a favourable wind (Coxe, iii. 368).

336. Mrs. Foley has not been identified.

337. Daniel Finch (1689–1769), son of the Earl of Nottingham.

338. Harley asked for the title Duke of Newcastle to be conferred on his son Edward (1689–1741) immediately after his marriage to the daughter of the defunct Duke in September 1713. He himself regretted his 'never enough to be lamented folly in mentioning to her Majesty the titles' (HMC *Portland* v. 466).

339. Anne retained a regard for Godolphin after his dismissal, and on his death 'seemed to be concerned'. Dartmouth suspected 'that there was an understanding between him and the queen to the last' (Burnet, vi. 143–4, note).

340. The truth of Hamilton's assertion is borne out by the autopsy report delivered on behalf of and in the presence of the other Royal physicians to the Council on 2 Aug. 1714, by Dr. Lawrence. However, the report indicates that the dissection was limited, for 'We can give no further account, being forbid making any other inspection than what was absolutely neccesssary for Embalming the Body' (*Guy's Hospital Gazette*, N.S. 24 (1910), 397–8).

APPENDIX A

The Queen and the Duchess, 1–18 January 1711

ON 1 January Sarah wrote a long letter to Hamilton which continued her story contained in the letter to him of 23 December (see p. xlii f.). This letter dealt with the interview with the Queen of 6 April and went up to and beyond Sunderland's dismissal.[1] In effect she told Hamilton what he already knew but the form of this letter accords closely with what was to become the *Conduct* and is consequently to be seen as virtually a summarizing of the end of the affair between the Queen and the Duchess. None the less, Sarah tried again to get to see the Queen with the Duke. She promised to behave herself for the future, but the Queen was unresponsive. Yet Sarah's letter of 1 January clearly occupied her for she proceeded to answer many of the points Sarah made in the letter, in a curiously self-justifying strain. Throughout the interview Hamilton tried to soothe the Queen by talking of the naturalness of self-vindication and hopefully suggesting that 'great Generosity' might bring the two together again. But the Queen was in no mood to hear offers of conciliation for she remembered too well Sarah's angry remonstrances on the occasion of the last interview. Sarah, in wishing that God should punish the Queen in this world or the next, ensured that her chances of reinstatement were remote. The Queen's memory filled in the gaps in Sarah's letters. The diary entry for the 5th demonstrates the degree of alienation which not only existed at this stage but which obviously had existed during all Sarah's attempts to regain her former standing. Sarah's animosity towards Anne and Anne's obstinate recoiling from facing her once favourite companion must have at least contributed towards the climate which enabled the ministerial revolution of 1710 to be effected. Harley understood his Queen better than Sarah did. In the evening of the same day Hamilton reported to Godolphin and to the Duke who began to realize how much Sarah had said during 1710 that he had not known about. He was, says Hamilton, extremely angry at his wife's outburst and must have seen disaster in the sense that the Queen was resurrecting a quarrel of many months ago. The Queen was gratified to hear of the Duke's anger and Hamilton urged the Duke (on the 6th) to attempt to ease the Queen, preparatory to the Duchess's owning her faults by letter. This

[1] Blenheim MSS. G-I-8 (fair copy). Another copy exists in Mary Cowper's hand (Panshanger MSS. D/EP F. 207). This latter copy adds a postscript: 'I write ye Inclos'd in such hast, yt I have taken no Copy of it, & some time or other, I wd have one because, you know nothing must be Omitted in my famous History I hope I shall see you to morrow night.'

appears once again to have been Hamilton's idea, and it was to lead to the interview of the Duke with the Queen of 17 January. The Queen on the 8th said in the same breath that she would keep Sarah in 'till it was over' and also that Harley would not press the Duke but that whether Sarah was in or not would not disgrace the Duke.

The old matter of the Queen's oath to Sarah was revived at this late stage, whether by Sarah or Hamilton is not clear. Hamilton talked of printing, arguably as a ploy to frighten the Queen and aid an uneasy truce. He argued that a peace between Harley and the Duke might forward a reconciliation with Sarah. The Queen flatly refused it. On relaying this reaction to the Marlboroughs, Sarah launched into a diatribe against ingratitude, quoted some of Anne's letters and said she knew things which could 'lose a Crown'. She was bitterly angry, whereupon Hamilton devised a scheme for reconciliation born out of optimism rather than a realistic view of the situation. He proposed a pact between Harley and the Duke for the purposes of the war effort; a bringing together of Sarah and Anne firstly by letter, secondly by the Duke's intercession, and, finally, by Sarah seeing the Queen; thirdly, and most optimistically, a reunion between Sarah and Abigail. Hamilton here saw that things were almost at an end and the oath still worried him greatly. On the 12th he read to the Queen some annotations on the 15th Psalm and on Ezekiel regarding an oath. The Queen's defence, as ever, was that circumstances and events had lessened the force of the promise. That the impending dismissal was in the Queen's mind is underlined by her comments to Hamilton on 13 January, where she recalled that Queen Mary wished to have Sarah dismissed. At this time she was fearful that the Duke might lay down but, says Hamilton, had been told that the Duke's ambition would keep him in. The oath concerned her sufficiently to have taken a Bishop's opinion, however. Hamilton on the 15th read the Bishop of Norwich's opinion and also gave the Queen the view of the Bishop of Bangor which he had written down (see Appendix C, p. 122). It was on the 15th that the Queen told Hamilton it was known that Sarah wrote to her and also that he had seen the letters. Hamilton denied ever having told anyone and gave her a letter from Sarah. He was still trying to persuade the Queen to keep Sarah until the Duke went out but the Queen decided that for Sarah to keep her places and not attend was a ludicrous state of affairs. On the evening of the 16th Hamilton made his last bid to reconcile the Queen and Sarah. He replied to Sarah's letter of the 15th and asked her to frame a letter of apology and duty to the Queen which might be used as the first stage of his three-point plan for the reunion (see above). Sarah replied:

I was in bed last night, before yr answer came to my letter, & a week's not time enough, to write wt you desire by nine a Clock. wch makes me send this by a footman, to waite till you come to ye backstairs, wt I had to say to you cannot be writt, & I will deffer it 'till 'tis convenient to you to come to me. I am very sorry to hear you have been so Ill, but I hope by this time yr pain is quite gone.[2]

On 17 January the long business drew to a close. Hamilton visited the Queen, presumably in the morning, and was told that if the Marlboroughs spoke of Sarah laying down that he was to give in to it but not to broach the subject himself. Hamilton told her how ill the Duke was. On the strength of the Queen's reaction, which the diary does not record, he wrote a note to the Marlboroughs saying 'I hav prepard the way by telling how ill m: L: duke was how deeply grievd about the affair that his expectation is from ye Q compassion to his Ds. I am of opinion to day is most fitting there seemd to be a great tenderness.'[3] Sarah noted after the dismissal that 'there was great reason to beleive this person was Employd by the q; to perswaid the D. of marl: to come that she might finish her design of puting me out, After hee had been with me the night before, & writt this leter in the morning by which I was to hope the queen would bee prevaild upon by lord marl: having expressed to this man great tendernesse'.[4] Sarah wrote her letter of humility, the Duke took it with him, and the Queen asked for the gold key. Sarah felt that Hamilton had been used by the Queen to effect the dismissal, but it is equally the case that Hamilton had, perhaps desperately, acted on his own behalf on the night of the 16th and had made his own interpretation of the Queen's feelings on the morning of the 17th. Going to the Queen on the 18th, Hamilton was told that the Duke had not been so 'tender' as might have been expected and that he had asked for and been given a fortnight to prevail on Sarah to lay down. Accordingly, he was told not to visit the Duke and Duchess unless they wrote. Hamilton sent an excuse. He was told on the 19th that the Duke had brought the key the previous evening.

The precise circumstances of what happened have never been made clear. According to Coxe[5] and all published accounts, the interview on 17 January consisted of the Queen's demanding the key within three days, and, on Marlborough's pleading for ten days, cutting the time to two days. The Duke went home and Sarah flung the key on the floor.[6] Yet the diary insists that the Duke brought the key on the 18th and not on the 17th. The story is made clear in a draft of the *Conduct* which shows that there were in fact two interviews, one on the 17th and another on the 18th. The duke (on the 17th)

waited upon her to represent to her, what she her self had been so sensible of before, the mischief this would be to her own affairs . . . However all the arguments he could make use of produc'd no other answer than this, that she must have

[2] Panshanger MSS. D/EP F. 207 (Mary Cowper's hand).

[3] Blenheim MSS. G-I-8. This is the only surviving note of Hamilton's to the Marlboroughs.

[4] Ibid., Sarah's hand, endorsing Hamilton's letter.

[5] iii. 175–7.

[6] Dartmouth's note to Burnet, VI. 33.

the Key . . . The next day I think the Duke of Marlborough went again to the Queen to complain of another strange step that had been taken to lessen his authority in the army, by disposing of three Commissions, without taking the least notice of it to him . . . But the Queen . . . could think of nothing else to say but that she could not talk to him about any thing 'till he had brought her the key; wch was the more ridiculous because this was a day or two before the time wch she her self had fix'd for it. Upon this I perswaded him to go again and carry it to her immediately, wch accordingly he did, and put an end to this matter.[7]

[7] Blenheim MSS. G-I-9, 'Memorandums for Mr. Hutchenson', pp. 33–4.

APPENDIX B

Hamilton's Scottish Circle

HAMILTON as an expatriate Scot wrote to his relatives and friends north of the border frequently and two little-used manuscript collections offer a vivid picture of the man and his times.[1] He was often called upon as a man of influence to help place younger relatives in a good position, to do favours for members of various more remote branches of the family and his efforts provide a useful commentary on his activities in London. His half-sister, Anna, had married David Boswell of Auchinleck whose son, James, married Lady Elizabeth Bruce. James and Elizabeth were the grandparents of Dr. Johnson's biographer who, later in the century, entertained the idea of writing a biography of Sir David.[2] There has survived a long series of letters of Hamilton's to James and Elizabeth Boswell ranging from 1696 to 1721, centrally about domestic family business but also giving more direct information about Hamilton's movements and his attempts to help his Scottish relatives.[3] Thus on 20 September 1696 James Boswell wrote from Leyden to ask Hamilton's advice about studies, diet, and a good physician in case of illness, thus beginning a friendship which was to go deeper than family obligation.[4] When James returned from Leyden, Hamilton made efforts to secure him an appointment via Lady Overkirk, a distant relative.[5]

Hamilton's status as a royal physician ensured that his aid would be requested on various occasions. Thus his kinsman, the third Laird of Dalzell, received a request dated 5 September 1713 from a friend asking him to introduce by letter one William Pettigrew, an 'Apothecary Surgeon' to Hamilton in order to place Pettigrew as a surgeon's mate on an East India ship or with 'some eminent Surgeon'. The writer adds a postscript in which he explains that 'The reason why I give you this trouble is because I reckon it will be my Nephew's great advantage to be under Sir David's ayd a person not only eminent as a physician, But whose name is savoury

[1] These are: letters to the family of Hamilton of Orbiston and Dalzell, bound up in 17 vols. in 1870, Motherwell Public Library; and Papers of James Boswell, Beinecke Rare Books Library, University of Yale, Talbot Papers (uncatalogued), especially Inventories 2 and 6.

[2] *Private Papers*, op. cit., vol. 12, p. 67; 21 Oct. 1776. There is nothing among the Boswell Papers to indicate that Boswell ever entered upon this undertaking.

[3] *Boswell Papers*, Talbot Papers, Inventory no. 2, p. 5, 51 letters.

[4] James's letter is in his Account Book kept in Holland, 1695–7 (*Boswell Papers*, c. 338, pp. 8–9). Throughout the rest of David Hamilton's life, he constantly sent to James in Scotland long letters concerning religious belief and the consequences of duty.

[5] *Boswell Papers*, letter to James Boswell (28 Dec. [?]).

as a serious and solid christian over all Brittain'.[6] Hamilton took these matters seriously. The diary for 3 July 1714 records his presenting a charitable petition from a Scots lady directly to the Queen, whilst in 1716 he attempted zealously to help a certain Alexander Murray, though the details of the outcome are unknown. Hamilton wrote to Murray to assure him that he would use his influence and that he would be glad

to have a memoriale wherby the expectation of your estate may be layd aside and so soon as I hav lookd over what you trusted me with Ile send them to you The detaile you gave me of your own affair is a respect and a confidence that I shall not forgett and shall never Use but for your honour and to serve you.[7]

Hamilton clearly is to attempt to help Murray probably as one who had access to the Prince but the exact nature of the promise is not clear. Murray's name occurs twice more in connection with Hamilton, once urging the Laird of Dalzell to visit London to see Sir David[8] and again in a letter written after Hamilton's death by his younger son, David,[9] who because of the death of his brother, Thomas, was left to sort out his father's affairs. In this letter of 6 March 1722 David confesses:

I was perfectly unacquainted wth. the Affair you mentiond in your Letter; I should be glad you'd perticularise the nature of Mr. Murrys Debt & the Method of coming att it for to speak the Truth my Father left that matter not quite so clear as I could have wisht wch. I impute to the hurry of Business he was always in engag'd in [*sic*] . . .[10]

More clearly documented is Hamilton's favour in 1716 to his brother's son, Archibald. Archibald Hamilton wrote to his father, the Laird, from Leyden on 12 June 1716 to say that Sir David had sent him news of the Laird's affairs via a letter to his own son, Thomas, '& at the same time hearing that I was to Go to paris asked to know if a Letter from him to my Lord Stairs wold do me any Service; since you are so Generous as to allow me to Go to france Ile write him a Letter of thanks & accept of His kind proffer'.[11] Hamilton subsequently wrote to the Earl on 24 July.[12] By November Archibald was back in London for his uncle wrote to him via David Hamilton's house.[13] And by January 1717, Archibald had taken chambers in

[6] *Orbiston Letters*, iv. f. 60.

[7] Edinburgh University Library, MS. La. II. 511. The letter is endorsed 'Sir David Hamilton . . . to the Prince . . . his first letter to me Alexr. Murray dated April 14 1716'.

[8] *Orbiston Letters*, v, f. 94. Murray to Archibald Hamilton (who subsequently became fourth Laird). The letter is undated.

[9] David had taken his B.A. at Oxford in 1721 and then matriculated as a student at Leyden on 29 May 1721 (Innes Smith, op. cit., p. 106). He presumably returned to England on his father's death, some three months later.

[10] *Orbiston Letters*, iv, f. 125. To Archibald Hamilton, who oversaw Hamilton's will and testament.

[11] Ibid., f. 163.

[12] Ibid., f. 168.

[13] *Orbiston Letters*, iv, f. 180 (15 Nov. 1716).

Edinburgh to begin his practice of the law, and he was insistent upon his obligations to Sir David. Writing to his father on 6 January he hopes that his father will

> write to Sir David & thank him for all his kindnesses to me & tell him that I flatter you with a belife that he wants to see you, (& tell him) that its impossible to think but that you have a Great inclination to see so near a relation, & one to whom you have been so much oblidged, & send him all the private news for God Sake dont neglect to write to him, your delaying writing so Long when I was at London, vex'd me so much, that it Gave me the jaundice . . .[14]

There was one other relative of Hamilton's who owed him no less than his life. As an ardent dissenter, Hamilton frequently prayed that England might avoid 'the yoke of Popery'.[15] At the time of the 1715 Rebellion, his principles and family loyalties were severely strained when he found that a kinsman, Robert, Earl of Carnwath, had been sent to the Tower on a charge of high treason for alleged complicity in the insurrection.

Between the impeachment and the sentence Hamilton spent a great deal of time attempting to obtain clemency for Carnwath. The most intense activity on Carnwath's behalf took place in February 1716.[16] Mary Cowper noted in her diary on 16 February that 'Sr. David Hamilton had a letter from my Ld Carwath [*sic*] who is his Second or third Cousin desiring him to come & speak to him, he has had leave & is gone to night'.[17] It transpired that '(3) [the Princess] had a great mind to save (171) [Carnwath] She has desird me to get (172) [Hamilton] to go to him & speak to him to Lay some ſoundation wth (1) [the King] to save him but I believe he wont but will persist in saying he knows nothing'.[18] On the 22 February Mary came out from the Princess and '(172) follow'd me, & brought me a letter for (3) from (171) . . . She took it & was much mov'd in reading it & wept, & sd he must say more to save himself. bid (172) go to him again & beg of him for Gods sake to save himself by confessing . . . I sent for (172) & gave him ye Orders . .'[19]

It was known that Carnwath had seen the Pretender in early 1714 and the basis of the plea for clemency was presumably that that meeting and the 1715 uprising were not specifically connected. Carnwath was eventually persuaded to give details of the meeting with the Pretender to Hamilton and '(171) followed (310) [Mary Cowper] to (3)'s house, where he gave (310)

[14] Ibid., f. 195.

[15] *Boswell Papers*, letter to James Boswell (1 Nov. 1715).

[16] Carnwath was impeached for high treason on 19 Jan. and sentenced to death on 9 Feb.

[17] Mary Cowper, Diary, f. 29.

[18] Ibid., f. 30 (20 Feb.). Hamilton's comments are contained in a letter to Mary Cowper, Panshanger MSS. D/EP F. 200.

[19] Mary Cowper, Diary, f. 31.

a letter from (171) to (172) confessing ye Conversation wth (666) [the Pretender] wch letter (310) has in keeping having show'd it to (3)'.[20] The next day Mary wrote that 'Sr. David Hamilton came to me & told me he had been wth my Ld Carnwath who knew nothing of his reprieve till eight a Clock this morning'.[21] Carnwath remained in the Tower for some time after this. On 25 February Hamilton was refused admission to the Tower, for 'they are more strictly kept since ye Escape'.[22] A letter survives of Carnwath to Mary Cowper (26 June 1716) thanking her for all she has done.[23] There is a revealing addition to the Carnwath affair by Mary Cowper's daughter, Lady Sarah Cowper, when she was at an assembly given by Lady Strafford, some time after the death of both parents. A gentleman came to her and paid his respects to her and to the memory of her parents 'with great Warmth, but much Incoherence & such an Air of Wildness, that I concluded him to be a Mad-Man, till upon his leaving me I ask'd Mrs. Caesar . . . who he was, & she told me Ld Carnwath. She said, he had been so terrified with the Fears of Death, that he had never since his Release, recover'd his Spirits, & always appear'd fluster'd tho' he was not Mad'.[24]

In the last three years of his life Hamilton's correspondence decreased. He wrote to Archibald Hamilton on 3 May 1718 expressing a hope that he and his father would visit him in London soon. There is a hint that he is not well for he alludes to the difficulty in writing letters by way of apology.[25] In the same letter he asks for a note to be delivered speedily concerning his coat of arms for the 'reason is about what crest I shall choose to my chariot, which I shall hav now ye end of ye month, & what I do now will be a foundation for the children to go on'.[26] Archibald Hamilton did go to London and on his proposing to return, he informed his father that he was bringing letters from David Hamilton to 'som of his particular friends, as well as my Self, which will abundantly Show his Inclinations and kind indeavours in my favours'.[27] There are no other surviving letters between Hamilton and his relations in Scotland.

[20] Mary Cowper, Diary, ff. 31–2 (23 Jan.). The letter is contained in Panshanger MSS.D/EP F. 200.

[21] Ibid., f. 32. This was in fact only a temporary respite. The sentence was altogether remitted under the Act of Indemnity.

[22] Ibid., f. 33. Hamilton confirmed this in a letter to Mary (Panshanger MSS. D/EP F. 200).

[23] Ibid.

[24] Ibid. D/EP F. 230, pp. 363–4.

[25] *Orbiston Letters*, v, f. 21.

[26] Ibid.

[27] Ibid., v, f. 98 (24 Sept. 1720).

APPENDIX C

The Contents List of the Original Diary

AMONGST the Blenheim manuscripts[1] is a twenty-four-page document in David Hamilton's hand. It is headed 'The Contents' and gives details of a version of the diary running to some 237 pages. It appears to be the original draft of the diary which was sent to Lord Cowper for his comments and advice (see p. xvii). Allowing for the fact that Hamilton's hand is larger than Mary Cowper's whose version provides the copy-text for this edition, there is a tantalizing amount of material which has, perhaps on Cowper's advice, been eliminated from Mary's copy. A study of the contents list indicates for example the omission of material which more fully demonstrates Hamilton's political leanings than the diary as it now exists (see contents, pp. 85–100, none of which has survived). Equally the contents reference (p. 24) to 'A Character of King George' did not find its way into the revised version. The list of contents, here transcribed exactly except that superior letters are brought down to the line, gives a clear idea of the scope and development of Hamilton's original draft of his diary and the process through which it passed in becoming the extant version.

The Contents

The immediate Occasion of the Queen's death, prov'd to be, the translation of the Gouty Humour from Her Knee and Foot upon Her nerves and Brain — 1

The Cause of this translation was disquiet of Mind — ibid

All this prov'd from Her Majesties own Authority — 2

The Queen alwayes well when she is easy in Her Mind — ibid

why the after-part of Her Life is loaded with reflections — 3

A Second proof that uneasyness of Mind was the Cause of the Translation — ibid

I caution Her Majesty against disquiet and she receives the Advice with thankfulness — 4

My Ld Godolphin then Treasurer comes to me and enquires of the Queen's Health — ibid

my reply to him and his answer to me — ibid

[1] F-I-16.

He promises to do his utmost to keep the Queen easy 5
I told Her Majesty what happen'd with my Ld Godolphin and she desires me to go on ibid
My Ld Godolphin acts the part of a kind Friend as well as that of a Minister of State ibid

He expresses great pleasure in keeping Her Majesty Quiet 6
The Queen orders me to discourse my Ld Godolphin about keeping Her quiet ibid
the Reason my Ld Marlborough absents from Court 7
The Queen tells me she is under great vexations ibid
Sacheverel's Affair occasions disquiet to her Majesty and Her opinion, about his punishment ibid
The Queen asks me if the Minds of the people are more easy 8
Endeavours to impress the Queen against Ld Godolphin 9
The Estrangement between the Queen and the Dutchess of Marlborough come to great height ibid
and the reasons thereof ibid
The Queen commands me to Speak to my Ld Godolphin, to influence the Dutchess to Make her submissions ibid
The Queen believing that the Dutchess govern'd Ld Godolphin committs the Affair to me 10

The Duke of Shrewsbury's coming in owing to the Estrangment between the Queen and Dutchess of Marlborough 10
The Queen not fully resolv'd to part with the Dutchess 11
The Bait with wch Her Majesty was intangled to change the Ministry 12
The Queen unwilling to part with my Ld Godolphin orders me to see if I cou'd bring him off from the Dutchess ibid
his answer to me ibid
My Ld Godolphin is of Opinion that the preferment of Mrs. Massam shou'd be Her Majesties own deed 13
My first interview with the Dutchess of Marlborough, with what pass'd therin 14

I told the Queen that the Fear of the City, was the Loss of Ld Godolphin 15
The Dutchess of Marlborough with me at my own House 16
The Narrative of what pass'd between us ibid

The people uneasy about the dissolution of the parliament 19
The Dutchess of Marlborough in passion about my Ld Sunderland's being put out 20
My Lady Marlborough designs to print ibid
The Methods I propos'd to the Queen to prevent Her printing 21
I caution the Queen against being too open to a Favourite from my Lady Marlborough's Behaviour ibid
Ld Godolphin approves of My Methods of dismissing the Dutchess ibid
My Advice to the Queen about the advancing of Money 22
Mr Wards of Opinion that the Tories cou'd not answer the Funds ibid
Her Majesty reads Lady Marlborough's Letter to me, wch reflects on the Queen and Her Ministry 23
A Character of King George 24
The Queen's Opinion of the Letter 25

I told the Queen that people said she was for the pretender 26
The Queen's Answer to the Commissioners of the Bank who came to supplicate Her not to Make any Change of Ministry ibid
The Ministry's gradual pressing Her Majesty, the occasion of future Changes 27
I told the Queen what pass'd in Conversation with the Dutchess about My Ld Godolphin's dismission 28
The Queen told me that she had desir'd the Dutchess not to come to Her and desir'd me to hear what she said 2
She mentions what Ld Marlborough had write to Her 30
The Queen says Ld Godolphin is too apt to believe whisperers ibid

The Clergy's Address from the Country
much taken Notice of 31
My Endeavours to keep up the Queen's
Honour ibid

The Dutchess imparts to me a great
Secret 32
wch I communicated to the Queen ibid
The Queen's Answer ibid
My discourse with Her Majesty
about the Dissolution of the parliament 33
The people afraid of the pretender for
two Reasons ibid
I press'd my Ld Cowper's Staying in
by orders from the Queen 34
His Answer to me ibid
Ld Chancellour gives up the Seals 35
The Queen not to be accused for In
sincerity, or Contradiction 36
My Ld Cowper's reasons for laying
down wch I imparted to the Queen 37
Her Majesty designs to send for Dr. Bradford 38
The Queen orders me to write to Her
at Windsor, but not to sign My Name ibid
I told Mr. Harley that people said he
wou'd learn the Queen to Equivocate 39
My Conversation with the Dutchess
of Marlborough in wch she reflects
upon the Duke of Somerset 40
The Dutchess of Marlborough's Letter
to me wch I read to the Queen 41
She Says Mr St John encourages the
Author of the Examiner, and she endeavours
to excuse Her-Self from the Imputations of the
Examiner 42
She says she will be forc'd to print
for Her own Justification 43
She Sends me the Observatour 45
The Queen's Opinion of the Dutchess
after she had read this Letter 46
The Dutchess of Marlborough asks
My Advice about Her going to Court 47
My Endeavours to impress the Queen well
as to Lady Marlborough ibid
The Queen complains that the Duke of
Marlborough is become ill natur'd 48

My Letter to the Dutchess wch the Queen
saw ibid
My Advice to the Dutchess 49
The Queen orders me to keep a
Copy of my Letter to the Dutchess 50
The Dutchess reflects on the Queen's
Speech and upon the Address of the Commons 51
She says in Her Letter that it is much
better to be wicked than Good ibid
She gives a Character of Mr Prior 52
The Queen said, the Dutchess's
passionate Temper Makes Her receive
ill Impressions before she knows the
Truth of any Thing 53
The Dutchess says that Her Intentions
are that Ld Marlborough shou'd not
serve any more 55
She reflects in Her Letter upon the
Duke of Argyle 56
She reflects bitterly upon the three
Secretarys of State 57
The Queen is positive, never to see
the Dutchess more. 58
The Queen order'd me to insist
that she shou'd not inflame the Duke
at his coming over. 59
The Queen designs that the Duke
shou'd continue to serve if he wou'd be
submissive ibid
The Queen calls Cadogan a sad fellow 60
The Queen tells me that the Intire
Defeat of Spain was true 61
I told Her Majesty that it was only in
Her power to keep a Ballance 62
The Dutchess complains that the
Queen has never given her any
Reasons, for Her Change 63
The Queen complains of the Dutchess's Inveteracy
against Mrs. Massam. 64
as also of her Saying Shocking Things 65
The Dutchess endeavours to justify
Her self in a Letter 66
She says she made the Queen
put out Ld Keeper Wright 68
She says she made the Queen
Take in Ld Sommers and Ld Orford 69

She excuses her Saying, Shocking Things 70
The Queen orders the Dutchess to lay what she has to say in writing before Her 72
I told the Dutchess that she had try'd to make the Queen Easy with her but in an unbecoming Manner 73
I told the Dutchess that if she had not continu'd her ill behaviour, and had not said shocking Things she might have recover'd the Queen's Kindness 76

The Queen said, that the Dutchess had no Hand in bringing in, Ld Cowper, Ld Sommers, nor Ld Orford 78

The Queen told me that the Dutchess had said as much to Her-self and afterward in Company, as that she lied ibid
The Queen said that Montague was just like her Mother 79
The Queen orders me to go to Ld Godolphin and take his Opinion as to the Affair in Spain 80
His opinion, how to retrive the Misfortune happen'd in Spain 81
The Queens tells me that Ld Marlborough had been very humble 82
The Duke of Marlborough's Reasons to me, why the war is more difficult now than before. 83
I told the Queen of Ld Marlborough's great Affection to Her ibid
Mr Harley endeavours to undermine the Constitution, and remove Ld Godolphin 85
The Torries endeavour to persuade the Queen That the Duke of Marlborough aims at the Crown 87
Mrs Massam willing to raise Her-Self at the Expence of her patroness 88
Mr Harley alwayes preferrs his own Interest to every Thing else ibid
The Queen impos'd upon by the Torries 89
The Torries poyson the Minds of the people ibid
The paper and pulpit war renew'd with great Heat 90
The Torries give Notice to the French King of the Divisions in England ibid

My Ld Godolphin's great Integrity 91
The Duke of Shrewsbury's Character 92
He enters into a Conspiracy against King William 93
He is forced to Marry Donna palliotti ibid
He carrys on the Designs of the pretender ibid
The Archbishop of york prepares The Queen for what was to follow 94
The disorders in England make the King of France break off his Treaty of peace with the Confederates 95
The Allies make applications to the Queen, against the Change of the Ministry. 96
The Queen by the Instigation of Mr. Harley incens'd against the Allies changes the whole Ministry 97
The Methods the Torries took to dissolve the parliament 98
Mr. Harley endeavours to amuse the Court of Hanover 99
The greatest part of the peers of Scotland for the pretender 100
The Dutchess of Marlborough tells me that Argyles Instalment is stop'd for want of Money 101
Secretary Glanvill sends his Man to do Business with Ld Marlborough ibid
I told the Queen that the Dutchess promis'd not to medle any more with politicks 102
The Queen tells me that the Dutchess has mention'd in Her Letters what she did and said, but not what the Dutchess Herself did and said 103
My reply to the Queen, and Her Answer to me, about the Dutchess ibid
The Duke of Marlborough angry with the Dutchess for having spoke so to the Queen 105
My speeches to the Queen in behalf of the Duke and Dutchess of Marlborough 106
The Queen says Her oath was conditional, on the Dutchess's behaviour ibid
I told the Duke and Dutchess what had pass'd between me and the Queen 107
The Dutchess Answer to me ibid
My scheme for a Reconciliation 109

The Queen tells me she is easy in that promise because of the Dutchess's ill behaviour 112
The Bishop of Norwich's opinion of the Queen's Oath. ibid
The Dutchess desirous to refer the whole Affair to a clergy-man 114
She desires only to stay in till my Ld Marlborough be put out 116
The Queen's answer to that proposal ibid
The Bishop of Bangor's Opinion of the Case 117
A most harsh and bitter saying of the Dutchess's to the Queen 120
The Queen complains of the Duke of Marlborough 121
The Duke brings the Key ibid
The good Effects of my Advice to the Queen ibid
The Queen's Favour to the Dutchess of Marlborough the great occasion of the Duke's Success. 122
The lessons I presented to Her Majesty, from My Lady Marlborough's Conduct 123
Dr Kennett's Opinion of the promise 124
The Dutchess by giving up the Key renounces her Title to the promise 126

The Queen's conversation and mine about the Dutchess of Shrewsbury 127
The Queen's Answer to one who ask'd how he shou'd vote ibid
The Convocation taken off from Hereditary Right and passive Obedience, and order'd to fix their Thoughts against Atheism and Immorality 128
The Duke of Marlborough's sharp Repartee to the Dutchess 129
My Conversation with the Duke of Marlborough before his departure for Flanders 130
The Queen's Opinion of Mr. Harley 131
I caution the Queen against Roman Catholicks 132
I propos'd to the Queen to have some of the Family of Hanover here 133
My Discourse with the Queen about the Bishop of Salisbury, Ld Cowper, and the pretender. 134
The Electour of Hanover's Answer to Ld Rivers. 135

THE CONTENTS LIST OF THE ORIGINAL DIARY

My Ld Cowper's Opinion about the peace	136
The Reason why Mr. Harley fail'd the 2d day in voting the Address with Advice to the Queen	137
Reflections on the Queen's Speech	ibid
The Reason why people said the Queen equivocated	139
The Reason why Ld Cowper laid down	140
Ld Nottingham for the Occasional Bill with my discourse with the Queen about it	141
My Advice to the Queen about the Ministry	142
The Queen's good Temper	143
Ld Harvey's Opinion of the Twelve Lords	144
My Advice to the Queen how to govern Her-self as to partys	145
A particular person's Opinion about the twelve Lords	146
My conversation with the Queen about the twelve Lords	147
I told the Queen what people said as to Her Affection to Favourits	148
My discourse with the Queen about the Dutchess of Somerset	ibid
The Queen orders me to speak to Ld Cowper about the Dutchess of Somerset's staying in.	150
The Duke of Somerset's Reasons why the Dutchess shou'd not stay in	151
My Advice to the Queen, that she shou'd not be so much influenc'd by Her Favourite	152
The Duke of Somerset condescends to the Dutchess's staying in	156
They begin to bespatter the Dutchess of Somerset	157
Her Majesty declines to read the Windsor prophecy	158
The Queen's Opinion of Dr Swift	159
My Conversation with the Queen about the Bill for Toleration in Scotland	160
My Discourse with the Queen about the Reformation of Manners	ibid
Reasons why people are afraid of the Pretender	162
The Queen's Discourse with me about, St John's being at the play with the pretender	165
Ld Cowper's discourse with me about the pretender and the Cessation of Arms	167

I told the Queen what Ld Cowper said about the pretender 169
The Queen's Opinion of Ld Cowper 170

Arguments, that the pretender is not the Real Son of King James the Second 171
Her Majesties kind Expression to me 173
The Dutchess of Somerset too reserv'd 175
The true signs of Friendship. 176
My Ld Cowper's Opinion concerning duelling 178
My discourse with the Queen, about the suitableness of the Dutchess of Somerset's Friendship 183
The Queen compar'd to King Asa and the gouty Foot. 185
What the Queen said about the Bishop of Salisbury ibid
Auditor Harley desirous to releas the Galley Slaves 187
Sr Richard Vivian's Opinion about the pretender communicated to the Queen 188
Polignac made Cardinal, by the Nomination of the pretender ibid
what people said of My Ld Dorset's and the Duke of Kent's conversation with the Queen. 191

I told the Queen what had happen'd between L H: and me 192
The Queen approves of my Answer to him ibid
I advis'd the Queen to give some proof, to the people of Her not being for the pretender.
people suspicious of Harley's designs, 193
as If he was for the pretender. 194
What she said of Ld Cowper 195
I propose to the Queen a way how to remove the Notion of Whig and Tory 196
Swift preferr'd by the Duke of Ormond, and not by the Queen. ibid
The Things that disquiet the Queen 197
why the Queen did not satisfy the people at all Times 199
The Queen's Opinion of the Bishop of Norwich ibid
The Queen uneasy about the Scots 200
My Conversation with Ld Marr ibid

The Queen's discourse with me
about Sr David Dalrymple 202
I communicated to the Queen what
was said against Ld Oxford 203
The Queen's Reasons for not desiring any of
The Family of Hanover, over. 204
The Queen shews great Kindness to
the Dutchess of Somerset ibid
My Son's saying, of the Duke
d'Aumont's present. 205
Objections against Her Majesties Speech ibid
My discourse with the Queen about
Lady Massam. 206
Ld Cowper's Opinion about the
proceedings of the parliament 207
I discours'd about Lady Mary Cochran. ibid
My discourse with the Dutchess
of Somerset about keeping the Queen quiet 208
Mr Caesar from Hanover and his
discourse with me. 209
The Queen desires me to consider
about Steel. 211
The Queen well satisfied with
what I did and said. 212
The Queen's opinion of the Duke
of Cambridge 214
Two signs of Bullingbrooks Influence
gaining Ground with the Queen
what she said of princess Sophia's death. 218
The Effects of My disquiet of
Mind, in hearing of my Mother's death 219
How Ld Oxford ruin'd his own Interest. 220
why Bourg desists from writing. 221
what mov'd me to think that Ld Oxford
was declining in the Queen's favour 222
The Queen's Answer to the
House's Address about the South-Sea. 222
The Reasons of the Queen's disquiet 223
The Queen misled by false Insinuations 224
why the Queen yielded to false Insinuations ibid
Ld Cowper's Excuse for not waiting
on the Queen. 225
My Conversation with Lady Massam. 226
The Queen's most kind discourse to me
about my faithfulness, and Integrity
towards Her. 227

The Electour of Hanover expresses his satisfaction with Bourg's Correspondence 229
The Queen promises that the change of Ministry shou'd not injure the Elector 230
The Queen resolves to send me to Hanover 231
My Errand thither ibid
The Queens great Confidence in me 232
Ld Oxford put out ibid
A true Account of the Queen's last sickness 233
A false Account of it, and the Reasons that mov'd people to say so 234
The Queen's Character 235
The Ministry's Conduct injures greatly the Queen. ibid
The Queen contrives to remove the Ministry, and therby to make Her Subjects Easy. 237

APPENDIX D

Godolphin's Advice to the Queen

GODOLPHIN'S memorandum to the Queen about the state of Spain after the battle of Brihuega is preserved in Bodleian MS. Rawlinson D. 924 f. 514.

My Lord Godolphin's Letter to
Sr David Hamilton, which was com-
municated to the Queen. [erased]

My Lord Godolphin's advice to the Queen directed
to Sir David Hamilton

Sir

I have here set down the substance of what I say'd to you last night, I am sorry it's so long, but I am always affray'd of not being intelligible, wch makes me apt to be too tedious.

The misfortune hapned in Spain, tho very great, is not wholly irrecoverable.

In order to it, King Charles must be encourag'd, without losing a moment's time, to reinforce Catalonia, where he has three places well fortify'd; Barcelona, Girona, and Tarragona, each of them capable of holding a two months siege, within which time, fresh forces may be sent both from Italy, England and Holland, not with intention to over-run Spain, by acting offensively, this misfortune haveing shewn, that that is not to be done, but that King Charles may be enabled to preserve his footing in Catalonia, till France be pressed on this side as to be obliged to give up Spain by treaty.

If the Queen's Ministers are hearty and sincere in their intentions, to support the Allyance, for the recovering of Spain, this misfortune in Spain, gives them such an occasion of shewing it so evidently to all the Allies, that when they see, the Queen does all that is possible to retrieve this blow, they will lose all that distrust, which is grown very much upon them, by the change of the ministry, and soon come to have the same confidence in her Majesties present ministers, as they had in the former, and when ever this trust and confidence is renewed, the credit will presently be restor'd with it, and indeed nothing else can ever restore it but that, wch at first rais'd it to so great a height in England, and that was the entire dependance wch all of the Allies had in the best and steadyest asistance of the Queen's Ministers, in the support of the war, till they cou'd bring France to a safe, as well as an honourable peace; and if the Queen's present ministers, upon this occasion will take such congrous [*sic*] measures, as are proper to restore that trust, and confidence in the Allies abroad there is no reason to doubt, but the credit will soon be restored with it.

BIBLIOGRAPHY

(*a*) MS. SOURCES

Alnwick Castle MSS.	Duke of Northumberland
Berkshire RO	Trumbull Additional MSS. 136/1

'Bills of Fare for their Royal Highnesses the Prince and Princess of Wales . . .' (1715–16), MS. in the possession of Kenneth Monkman, Esq.

Blenheim MSS.	Duke of Marlborough (Duchess of Marlborough, Arthur Mainwaring, David Hamilton: A-I-26; C-29; E-20, 25, 27, 29, 37; F-I-16; G-I-7, 8, 9, 10, 16)
BODLEIAN LIBRARY	
MS. Eng. poet. e. 50	Poem on Hamilton's Knighting
MS. Rawlinson, A. 289	Hamilton's appointment as second physician
MS. Rawlinson, D. 924	Godolphin/Hamilton's memo.
MS. Carte, 125	Thomas Carte
MS. Ballard, 21	Delaune to Charlett
MS. Ballard, 38	Bromley to Charlett
BRITISH MUSEUM	
Loan 29	Harley family
Additional MSS.	
9107	Godolphin to Marlborough
28101	Poem on Hamilton's Knighting
34223	Westmorland's Memoirs
40060	Poem on Hamilton's Knighting
47027	Helena le Grand
Stowe MSS.	
305	Poem on Hamilton's Knighting
Sloane MSS.	
3516	Elegy for Hamilton
4044	Hamilton letters
4059	Hamilton letters
4075	Hamilton letters
Lansdowne MSS.	
1014	White Kennett
1024	White Kennett
Churchill College, Cambridge	Drax MSS. (Marlborough to Erle)
Edinburgh, University Library	MS. La. II, 511 (Alexander Murray)
Guildhall Library	MS. 5686 (Hamilton's second marriage)
HERTFORDSHIRE RO	
Panshanger MSS.	
D/EP 33	Dame Sarah Cowper's Diary
,, 71–8	Earl Cowper's pocket diaries
,, 200	David Hamilton

D/EP 205	Mary Cowper's diary
„ 207	David Hamilton's diary
„ 229	Lady Sarah's copy of the diary
„ 230	Lady Sarah Cowper's papers
Huntingdon Library, California	Stowe MSS. (James Brydges)
Leicestershire RO	Finch MSS.
Motherwell Public Library	Hamilton of Dalzell Papers
Northamptonshire RO	Finch–Hatton MSS.
Prussian State Archives	Bonet to Frederick I
Public Record Office	Lord Chamberlain; State Papers Domestic; Sir John Cropley to Shaftesbury (30/24/20 and 21)

Royal College of Physicians, MSS. Annals (contemporary transcript vols. v–viii, 1682–1722)

St. Katherine Coleman, London, MS. Register Book (1666–1741): deposited at the parish church of St. Olave, Hart Street, London

Scotland, National Library	MS. 23. 2. 24. (Hamilton's knighting)
Scottish RO	Edinburgh Testaments, General Register House, Edinburgh (Hamilton's will, 1731)
Wiltshire RO	Todd, Christopher, Letter to Hamilton, MS. 79b/4
University of Yale	Papers of James Boswell, Beinecke Rare Books Library, University of Yale. (i) Talbot Papers, Inventory no. 2, Hamilton to James Boswell. (ii) Ibid., Inventory no. 6, Lady Overkirk to Elizabeth Boswell

(*b*) PRINTED BOOKS

Place of publication is London, unless otherwise stated

Anderson, John, *Historical and Genealogical Memoirs of the House of Hamilton* (Edinburgh, 1825)

Arkell, R. L., *Caroline of Ansbach* (1939)

Beattie, J. M., *The English Court in the Reign of George I* (Cambridge, 1967)

The bishop of London's seventh letter at the conference with his clergy held in the year 1686 (1690)

Bodleian Library, Nichols Newspapers

Bolingbroke, Henry St. John, *A letter to the Examiner printed in the year 1710*

—— *A letter to Sir William Windham* (1717)

—— *Letters and Correspondence . . . of Henry St. John, Lord Viscount Bolingbroke*, ed. G. Parke, 4 vols. (1798)

Boswell, James, *Private Papers of James Boswell from Malahide Castle*, ed. G. Scott and F. A. Pottle, vols. 12 and 14 (1931–2)

Boyer, Abel, *History of the Reign of Queen Anne digested into Annals*, 11 vols. (1703–13)

—— *The Political State of Great Britain*, 2nd edn., 8 vols. (1718)

Bradford, Samuel, *An exhortation to purity and peace . . . preach'd in the parish-church of St. Mary le Bow . . .* (1710)

British Museum, Burney Newspapers

BIBLIOGRAPHY

BURNET, Bp., *The new preface and additional chapter to the third edition of the Pastoral Care* (1712)

—— *Bishop Burnet's History of his Own Time*, 6 vols. (Oxford 1833)

Calendar of State Papers (Domestic)

Calendar of Treasury Books

Calendar of Treasury Papers

CAMPBELL, Lord, *Lives of the Lord Chancellors . . .*, 8 vols. (1845–7, 69)

CARSWELL, J., *The South Sea Bubble* (1960)

CHAMBERLAYNE, Edward, *Angliae Notitia: or the Present State of England*, 21st edn. (1704)

CHAMBERLAYNE, John, *Magnae Britanniae Notitia*, 21st edn. (1708); 23rd edn. (1710)

CHESTER, J. L., *The Parish Registers of St. Mary Aldermary, London, 1558–1754*, Harleian Soc. Publ., vol. 5 (1880)

CHURCHILL, Sarah, *An Account of the Conduct of the Duchess of Marlborough* (1742)

—— *Private Correspondence of Sarah, Duchess of Marlborough*, 2 vols. (1838)

CLARKE, Samuel, *Scripture Doctrine of the Trinity* (1712)

COBBETT, William, *The Parliamentary History of England*, 12 vols. (1806–12); vols. 13–36 (1812–20)

A Collection of the addresses which have been presented to the queen since the impeachment of the Reverend Dr. Henry Sacheverell (1710)

CONNELL, N., *Anne the Last Stuart Monarch* (1937)

COWPER, Lord, *The Private Diary of William, First Earl Cowper*, ed. E. C. Hawtry (Roxburgh Club, 1833)

—— *A letter to Isaac Bickerstaff Esq.: occasion'd by the Letter to the Examiner* (reprinted in Boyer, *Annals*, ix, Appendix, 71–90)

—— *History of Parties presented to George I* (printed in Campbell (see above))

COXE, Archdeacon, *Memoirs of the Duke of Marlborough*, new edn. rev. by John Wade, 3 vols. (1905–8)

The Cure of the Miliary Fever . . . By a Subject to Mithridates, King of Pontus (1751)

DAVENANT, Charles, *Essays upon the balance of power* (1701)

—— *A true picture of a modern Whig* (1701)

DEFOE, Daniel, *An Essay upon Public Credit . . .* (1710)

—— *The Banb - - - y Apes* (1710)

—— *Dr. Sacheverell's disappointment at Worcester*

—— *A New Map of the laborious and painful travels of our blessed high church apostle*

DICKINSON, H. T., *Bolingbroke* (1970)

DICKSON, P. G. M., *The Financial Revolution in England* (1967)

FORSTER, T., *Original letters of Locke, Algernon Sidney and Lord Shaftesbury* (1833)

FOSTER, J., *Alumni Oxonienses 1500–1714*, 4 vols. (1891–2)

—— *Alumni Oxonienses 1715–1886*, 4 vols. (1887–8)

FRASER. W., *The Earls of Cromartie, Their Kindred, Country and Correspondence*, 2 vols. (Edinburgh, 1876)

The French king's reasons against peace (1710)

FRESHFIELD, E., *Register Book of the Parish of St. Christopher le Stocks*, 2 vols. (1882)

GREEN, David, *Sarah Duchess of Marlborough* (1967)

—— *Queene Anne* (1970)

HAMILTON, David, *Disputatio Medica Inauguralis de Passione Hysterica* . . ., (Paris (?), 1686)

—— *The Private Christian's Witness for Christianity: In Opposition to the Notional and Erroneous Apprehensions of the Arminian, Socinian, and Deist of the Age* (1697)

—— *The Inward Testimony of the Spirit of Christ To His Outward Revelation. In Opposition to the Deist, Socinian and Prophane. Who deny both* . . . (1701)

—— *Tractatus Duplex Prior de Praxeos Regulis Alter de Febri Miliari* (1710) (translation 1737)

The Diary of John Hervey, First Earl of Bristol (Wells, 1894)

Letter-Books of John Hervey, First Earl of Bristol, 3 vols. (Wells, 1894)

Historical Manuscripts Commission, Portland MSS.; Westmorland MSS.; Stuart MSS.; Polwarth MSS.; Bath MSS.

HOLMES, Geoffrey, *British Politics in the Age of Anne* (1967)

—— *The Trial of Doctor Sacheverell* (1973)

HONE, C. R., *The Life of Dr. John Radcliffe 1652–1714* (1950)

HOPKINSON, M. R., *Anne of England* (1934)

HORN, D. B., *British Diplomatic Representatives 1689–1789* (Camden 3rd Ser., 1932).

HORWITZ, H. G., *Revolution Politicks* (Cambridge, 1968)

House of Commons Journals

HOUSTON, James, *Dr. Houstoun's Memoirs of his own Life-Time* (1747)

HUNTER, R., and MACALPINE, I., *Three Hundred Years of Psychiatry 1535–1860* (1963)

The justice and necessity of restraining the clergy (1715)

KENYON, J. P., *The Popish Plot* (1972)

LAMBERTY, *Mémoires pour servir à l'Histoire du XVIIIe siècle* (Hague, 1730)

A letter concerning allegiance, written by the Lord bishop of L - - - - n (1710)

A letter to a friend concerning the publick debts, particularly that of the navy (1711)

A letter to the good people of Great Britain (1710)

The Lockhart Papers (1817)

LUTTRELL, Narcissus, *A Brief Historical Relation of State Affairs from Sept. 1678 to April 1714*, 6 vols. (Oxford, 1857)

MACKY, John, *Memoirs of the Secret Services of John Macky, Esq.* (Roxburgh Club, 1895)

MATTHEWS, W. (transcr. and ed.), *The Diary of Dudley Ryder 1715–1716* (1939)

MICHAEL, W., *The Beginnings of the Hanoverian Dynasty* (1936)

MIEGE, Guy, *New State of England*, 6th edn. (1707)

MILLER, H. K., ROTHSTEIN, E., and ROUSSEAU, G. S., *The Augustan Milieu: essays presented to Louis A. Landa* (Clarendon Press, 1970)

Now or Never: or, a project under God to secure the Church of England in a congratulatory letter to the right honourable the earl of D . . . upon his late promotion. Ibid., 'By a well-meaning Tory, who is willing to clear the Church of England from Jacobitism'

POTTLE, F. A., and SCOTT, G., *Private Papers of James Boswell from Malahide Castle*, 18 vols. (privately printed, 1928–34)

Queries, Somers Tracts, xii. 168–70

The Record of the Royal Society of London, 4th edn. (1940)

SEDGWICK, R., *History of Parliament 1715–1754* (1970)

SKINNER, H. A., *The Origin of Medical Terms* (Baltimore, 1961)

SMITH, R. W. Innes, *English-Speaking Students of Medicine at the University of Leyden* (Edinburgh, 1932)

STRADA, Faminianus, *de Bello Belgico . . .* [*1555–90*], (Rome, 1632–47). *The History of the Low-Countrey Warres . . . written in Latin by Faminianus Strada; Englished by Sir Rob. Stapylton, Kt.* (1667)

STRICKLAND, Agnes, *Lives of the Queens of England*, 8 vols. (1851, 2)

SWIFT, Jonathan, *The Windsor Prophecy* (1711)

—— *The Examiner* (1710–11)

—— *Poetical Works*, ed. H. Davis (Oxford, 1967)

—— 'An Enquiry into the Behaviour of the Queen's last Ministry', *Political Tracts 1713–1719*, ed. H. Davis and I. Ehrenpreis (Oxford, 1953)

—— *The History of the Four Last Years of the Queen* (1758)

—— *The Correspondence of Jonathan Swift*, ed. H. Williams, 5 vols. (Oxford, 1963–5)

—— *Journal to Stella*, ed. H. Williams, 2 vols. (1948)

SYDENHAM, Thomas, *Tractatus de Podagra et de Hydrope* (1683). Swan's 1742 translation in COMRIE, J. D., *Selected Works of . . . Sydenham* (1922)

TEMPLE, Sir William, *Works*, 4 vols. (Edinburgh, 1754)

A Test offer'd to the consideration of the electors of Great Britain (1703)

THOMSON, Mrs., *Memoirs of Viscountess Sundon*, 2 vols. (1847)

A true list of the names of those persons committed to the several goals [sic] *in and about London and Westminster . . . on account of the tumult, &c. March the 1st, 1710*

The True Patriot Vindicated, or a justification of the late earl of Rochester (1711)

The Tryall of Dr. Henry Sacheverell (1710)

WALPOLE, R. (?), *A short history of the parliament* (1718)

The Wentworth Papers 1705–1739, ed. J. J. Cartwright (1883)

WILKINS, W. W., *Political Ballads of the Seventeenth and Eighteenth Centuries* (1860)

WOODWARD, Josiah, *An account of the rise and progress of the religious societies, in the City of London, etc. and of their endeavours for reformation of manners* (1701)

WYON, F. W., *The History of Great Britain during the Reign of Queen Anne*, 2 vols. (1876)

(*c*) ARTICLES

BROMLEY, J. S., 'The French privateering war', *Hist. Essays pres. to David Ogg*, ed. H. E. Bell & R. L. Ollard (1963)

BUCK, C. and DAVIES, G., 'Letters on Godolphin's Dismissal in 1710', *Huntington Lib. Quarterly*, 3 (1940), 225–42.

BURTON, I. F., 'The Committee of Council at the War-Office', *Historical Journal*, 4 (1961), 78–84

'Earl Coningsbie's History of Parties presented to King George the First', *Archaeologia*, 38 (1860)

HILL, B. W., 'The change of government and the "loss of the City", 1710–11', *Economic Hist. Review*, 24 (1971), 395–413

HOLMES, Geoffrey, 'The Hamilton Affair of 1711–1712: a crisis in Anglo-Scottish relations', *English Historical Review*, 77 (1962), 257–82

—— 'Harley, St. John and the death of the Tory party', in *Britain after the Glorious Revolution* (1969), pp. 216–37

—— and SPECK, W. A., 'The Fall of Harley in 1708 reconsidered', *English Historical Review*, 80 (1965), 673–98

HORWITZ, H. G., 'Comprehension in the later seventeenth century; a postscript', *Church History*, 3 (1965), 1–7

PLUMB, J. H., 'The organisation of the Cabinet in the reign of Queen Anne', *Trans. Royal Historical Society*, 5th ser. (1957), 137–57

Post-Mortem on the body of Queen Anne transcribed in the *Guy's Hospital Gazette*, N.S., 24 (1910), 397–8

ROBERTS, Philip, 'Swift, Queen Anne, and *The Windsor Prophecy*', *Philological Quarterly*, 49 (1970), 254–8

SNYDER, H. L., 'The Last Days of Queen Anne: The Account of Sir John Evelyn Examined', *Hunt. Lib. Quart.*, 34 (1971), 261–76.

INDEX

References to Queen Anne and Sir David Hamilton in the diary itself are not indexed, since they appear on virtually every page. They are fully indexed as regards the Introduction, Notes, and Appendices.

Address [from the clergy], 16
Anglesey, Arthur Annesley, 5th Earl of, 63
Anne, Queen, xvii–xxi, xxiii–xxix, xxxi–xxxii, xlvii, 112, 115–27; quarrel with Duchess of Marlborough, xxxii–xlv, 107–10
Antoninus, Marcus, xl–xli
Applebee's Original Weekly Journal, xxx n. 78
Arbuthnot, Dr. John, xxiii, 37, 60
Argyle, John Campbell, 2nd Duke of, 24, 85 n. 121, 119
Argyle, Duchess of, xxx
Ashburnham, Lady, 48

Bangor, John Evans, Bishop of, 28, 108, 122
Beck, J., 10, 37, 48
Bedford, Wriothesley Russell, 2nd Duke of, xx n. 16
Bedford, Duchess of, xx and n. 16
Bernstorff, Count Von, xxiv and n. 43
Bishop's letter to his Diocese, 16
Bolingbroke, Viscount, *see* St. John
Bolton, Charles Powlet, 2nd Duke of, xxix n. 72
Boswell, David, David Hamilton's brother-in-law, 111
Boswell, James, David Hamilton's nephew, xxi n. 24, 111 and n. 4
Boswell, James, David Hamilton's great-grand-nephew, xxi n. 20, xxiii n. 32, 111
Boyle, Henry, 17
Bradford, Samuel, D.D., 19, 22, 67, 118
Brihuega, battle of, 83 n. 106, 127
Bruce, Lady Elizabeth, wife of James, David Hamilton's nephew, 111

Cadogan, William, 21, 119
Caesar, Dr. Julius, 56, 59, 125
Carmarthen, Peregrine Osborne, Marquis of, xviii, 17, 33, 79 n. 77
Carmarthen, Elizabeth Harley, Lady, 59
Carnwath, Robert Dalzell, 5th Earl of, 113–14
Cavendish, Henrietta, daughter of the Duke of Newcastle, 54, 64
Chamberlain, Dr. Hugh, 48
Charles I, King, 44
Charles II, King, 43–4
Cheyne, Dr. George, xxvi, xxvii n. 62
Churchill, Anne, 15–16, 30
Churchill, George, 21, 27, 86 n. 131
Churchill, John, *see* Marlborough, Duke of
Churchill, Sarah, *see* Marlborough, Duchess of
Clarendon, Edward Hyde, 3rd Earl of, 61
Clarke, Samuel, D.D., 17
Clayton, Mrs., xxix
Cochran, Mary, Lady, 58, 62, 64–5, 112, 125
Coke, Thomas, 63
College of Physicians, London, xix and n. 7, xx–xxi and n. 23
Comprehensions, bill of, 20
Convocation, 30
Cotton, Mrs., 48
Cowper, William, 1st Lord, xvii–xviii, xxxi, xlii, 17–19 (resignation 1710), 22, 29, 31–4, 36, 37–40, 41, 43–5, 47, 49–56, 58–64
Cowper, Mary, Lady, xvii, xxiii n. 39, xxiv and n. 43, xxv n. 48, xxix–xxxi, xxxv n. 92, xlvii–xlviii, 30, 113–15
Cowper, Dame Sarah, xxii
Cowper, Sarah, Lady, xviii, xlvii–xlviii, 114
Crowley, Sir Ambrose, xxii

Daily Courant, 94 n. 217
Daily Post, xxiv, xxx n. 78
Dalrymple, Sir David, 56, 125
Danvers, Isabella, 48, 62
Davenant, Charles, 17
Delawarr, John West, 15th Lord, 29, 87 n. 147
Denmark, George, Prince of, Anne's husband, 4
Donnellen, Mrs., 59
Dorset, Lionel Sackville, 10th Earl of, 52, 124
Duc D'Aumont, 49, 57, 125
Dunkirk, 42

Erle, Thomas, 15
Essay upon Credit, the, 17
Evening Post, 42
Examiner, xxxix–xl, 49, 57, 118; *a letter to the*, 17
Eyles, Francis, 11
Ezekiel, 27, 108

Flying Post, 44, 49–50, 102 n. 297
Foyston, Mary, 57

George I, King, xviii, xxi n. 23, xxix, 68, 115, 117; Hamilton's petition to, xvii, xx, xxiii–xxiv, xxvii–xxix, xxxii; Elector of Hanover, 20, 31–2, 34, 42, 53, 60–1, 64–7, 122, 126
Gloucester, William, Duke of, son of Queen Anne, 3, 25
Godolphin, Sidney, 1st Earl of, xviii, xxxi, xxxviii, 15–16, 19, 21, 23, 25, 48–9, 51, 56, 65, 73 n. 30, 115–17, 120–1, 127; Lord Treasurer, 4–7, 9–11, 13; dismissal, 14, 76 n. 57; and Duchess of Marlborough, xxxiii–xxxv, xliii, 8–9, 11, 107
Granville, Anthony Perenott, Lord of, 18
Granville, George, 24, 121

Hamilton, Anna, David Hamilton's sister, 111
Hamilton, Archibald, David Hamilton's nephew, xxiv, 112–14
Hamilton, Dr. David, physician to Queen Anne, biographical details, xvii, xix–xxiv; medical theory and practice, xx–xxi, xxv–xxx; political views, xviii, xxxi–xxxii; quarrel between Duchess of Marlborough and Queen Anne, xxxii–xlv, 107–10; Scottish circle, 111–14; diary, composition, xvii–xviii, xlvii–xlviii; diary, original contents, 115–26
Hamilton, David, the younger, xx and n. 12, xxiv and n. 47, xxxi n. 80, 112 and n. 9
Hamilton, Isobell, David Hamilton's mother, xix, xxi n. 24, 62, 125
Hamilton, James, David Hamilton's father, xix
Hamilton, James Douglas, 4th Duke of, 34
Hamilton, John, 47, 50
Hamilton, Thomas, David Hamilton's son, xx and n. 12, xxiii and n. 35, xxx–xxxi and n. 80, 57, 66, 112, 125
Hampden, Richard, 57
Hanover, George Augustus, Electoral Prince of, 60–1, 103 n. 310, 125
Hanover, Princess Sophia, Dowager Electress of, xviii, 61, 125
Harcourt, Simon, 1st Lord, 18, 34, 51, 89 n. 176
Harley, Abigail, xxviii
Harley, Edward, Auditor of the Imprest, 51, 124
Harley, Edward, Robert Harley's son, 64
Harley, Robert, 1st Earl of Oxford, xxxiii–xxxiv, xxxviii, 15, 17–19, 21, 24, 31–4, 36, 48, 51, 54–8, 60–5, 74 n. 39, 76 n. 55, 107, 118, 120–6; attempts to remove Hamilton, xxxi–xxxii; and Duke of Marlborough, 26–7, 108; attempted assassination, 44; the 12 lords, 91 n. 188; and the Duke of Cambridge, 103 n. 310; dismissal, 67
Harley, Sarah, wife of Edward, 52, 65
Harley, Thomas, Robert Harley's cousin, 61
Hertford, Algernon Seymour, Lord, 21, 54
Hervey, James, son of the Earl of Bristol, xxviii
Hervey, John, 1st Earl of Bristol, xxviii, xxx
Hervey, Lady, xxviii, xxx
Hervey, John, 1st Lord, 32, 36, 41, 49–50, 52, 55, 123
Hill, John, brother of Abigail Masham, 6
Hoadley, Benjamin, 17
Houstoun, Dr., *accoucheur*, 22 n. 32
Hume, Sir Gustavus, xxix n. 73
Hunsdon, William Carey, 8th Lord, 33, 89 n. 168

James II, King, 36, 124

Kennett, White, D.D., xvii n. 1, 29, 122
Kent, Henry Grey, 1st Duke of, 52, 73 nn. 23, 25, 124
Killigrew, Thomas, 43–4
Kingston, Evelyn Pierrepont, 5th Earl of, 55

Lane, Elizabeth, David Hamilton's second wife, xx–xxii
Lane, Sir Thomas, xx
Le Grand, Helena, xxii
Letter to the Freeholders, 20
Leyden, University of, xix and n. 6, xxiii, xxv, 66
Lister, Dr. Martin, xxviii
Louis XIV, King of France, 3, 31–4, 44, 53, 55, 120–1
Luttrell, Narcissus, xx

Maccartney, George, 45, 47
Mar, John Erskine, 6th Earl of, 55, 65, 124
Margaret, Duchess of Parma and Piacenza, 18
Marlborough, John Churchill, 1st Duke of, xxxii, xxxiv n. 91, 33, 37, 44, 62, 64, 73 n. 30, 116–17, 119–22; crisis over Essex regiment, 6, 71 n. 15; involved in wife's quarrel with Queen Anne, xxxvi–xliv, 12–13, 15, 20–31, 107–10
Marlborough, Sarah, Duchess of, estrangement from Queen Anne, xviii, xix, xxviii, xxxi–xlv, 4, 6–13, 15–16, 19–31, 35, 37, 40, 43, 107–10, 116–22; on Sunderland's dismissal, 12; on Godolphin's dismissal, 15, 76 n. 57; her dismissal, 29
Mary II, Queen, 3, 10, 25, 27–8, 57, 108
Masham, Abigail, Lady Masham, xliii–xliv, 6–7, 10, 13, 22, 24–5, 27, 40, 48, 51, 57–8, 64–5 67, 85 n. 127, 108, 116, 119–20, 125

INDEX

Maynwaring, Arthur, xxxvii and n. 103, 72 n. 16, 85 n. 128
Mead, Dr. Richard, 31
Millepedes, Spirit of, 4
Montague, John Montague, 2nd Duke of, 23
Montague, Lady, 15–16, 23, 30, 120
Montrose, James Graham, 1st Duke of, xxi
Moore, Arthur, 54, 62
Murray, Alexander, 112

Navy Bills, 21
'Necessitous Lords', the, 29
Newcastle, John Holles, 1st Duke of, xxxi n. 83, 34
Newcastle, Margaret, dowager Duchess of, 54
Noailles, Cardinal, 32
Noble, Richard, 51
Norwich, Charles Trimnell, Bishop of, 28, 55, 108, 122, 124
Nottingham, Daniel Finch, 2nd Earl of, 34, 50, 90 n. 183, 123
Now or Never, 17

Observator, 118
Occasional Conformity Bill, 4th (1711), xxxi–xxxii, 34
Onslow, Sir Richard, 11
Orford, Edward Russell, 1st Earl of, 22, 119–20
Ormonde, James Butler, 2nd Duke of, 54, 124
Overkirk, Lady, 111
Oxford, Earl of, *see* Harley, Robert
Oxford, Oriel College, xx n. 12, xxiii

Perceval, Sir John, xxii
Piquebourg, Countess of, xxix
Polignac, Abbot of, 51, 124
Post Boy, xxiv, 42, 50, 91 n. 194
Poulet, John Poulet, 1st Earl, 33
'Pretender', *see* Stuart, James Francis
Prior, Matthew, 119
Psalm 15, 16, 27, 108
Pye, Lady, xxviii

Querie upon Querie, 16
Queries, 14, 77 n. 64

Radcliffe, Dr. John, xxvi, 31, 87 n. 151
Rheims, University of, xix, xxv, xxvii
Rialton, Lady, 15, 16, 23, 30
Richmond, Charles Lennox, 6th Duke of, xxi
Rivers, Richard Savage, 4th Earl of, 20, 31, 77 nn. 61–2, 122
Robethon, Jean, 48
Royal Society, the, xxi and n. 22
Ryder, Dudley, xxix n. 73

Sacheverell, Henry, D.D., 6–7, 17, 72 n. 19, 116
St. Albans, Charles Beauclair, 1st Duke of, xxix n. 72
St. John, George, 61
St. John, Henry, Viscount Bolingbroke, 24, 34, 43, 61–2, 67, 89 n. 176, 102 n. 294, 118, 123, 125
St. Katherine Coleman, London, xix, xxiv
Salisbury, Gilbert Burnet, Bishop of, 31–2, 50, 122, 124
'Scheme Lords', the, 29
Schulenberg, Matthias John, Baron, 60–1, 63, 65–7, 125–6
Schütz, Baron, 61, 103 n. 310
'Scots Lords', the, 29
Seafield, James Ogilvy, 1st Earl of, 55
Shadwell, Sir John, xxiii and n. 40, xxvii, 50
Short History of the Parliament, A, 58
Shrewsbury, Charles Talbot, 1st Duke of, xxxv, 8, 15, 29, 50, 73 n. 24, 116, 121
Shrewsbury, Duchess of, 29, 50, 121–2
Sloane, Sir Hans, xxiv–xxv and n. 48
Soissons, Olympia, Countess of, 37
Somers, John, 1st Lord, 22, 119–20
Somerset, Charles Seymour, 6th Duke of, 15, 21, 28, 37–40, 58, 118, 123
Somerset, Duchess of, 21–2, 37–41, 45–50, 53, 56–9, 123–5
South Sea Company, xxii and n. 32, 43, 63, 125
Stair, John Dalrymple, Earl of, 112
Starkie, Mary, David Hamilton's first wife, xix, xxii
Starkie, Major Philip, xix
Steel, 31, 59, 62, 125
Steele, Sir Richard, 44
Steingens, the Palatine Resident in London, 60–2, 64–6
Stewart, John, 29
Strada, Faminianus, 18, 80 n. 88
Strafford, Thomas Wentworth, Earl of, 97 n. 241
Strafford, Lady, 114
Stringer, Thomas, xxviii
Stuart, James Francis, 'the Pretender', xviii, 14, 17, 20, 31–2, 34, 42–4, 50–5, 57, 60–1, 65, 113–14, 117–18, 121–4
Sunderland, Charles Spencer, 3rd Earl of, xxxiv–xxxv, xxxvii, xlvii, 10–12, 33, 55, 117
Sunderland, Lady, 15–16, 23, 30–1
Swift, Jonathan, xxxv, xxxix, 40–1, 43, 47, 54, 76 n. 57, 91 n. 187, 93 n. 206, 123–4; *The Windsor Prophecy*, 40, 92 nn. 203–4, 123
Sydenham, Dr. Thomas, xxv–xxvii

Test of the Elections, 16
Tipping's Water, 57

Todd, Christopher, xxii
Trevor, Sir Thomas, 1st Lord, 51

Union of England and Scotland, Treaty and Act of, 3, 55, 93 n. 207
Utrecht, University of, xxiii, 66

Vivian, Sir Richard, 51, 55, 124

Wales, Caroline of Anspach, Princess of, wife of George II, xxiv, xxix–xxx and n. 77, xxxi, 82, 113
Ward, John, 13, 117
Weekly Journal or British Gazetteer, xxx n. 78
Weekly Journal or Saturday's Post, xxx n. 78
Westmorland, Thomas Fane, 1st Earl of, xxviii
Wharton, Thomas, Earl of, 63
Wilks, Mrs. Judith, 45
William III, King, 27, 37, 42, 121
Williamson, C., xxiv
Willis, Dr. Thomas, xxvi
Wilmote, Mrs., xxviii
Windsor Prophecy, The, *see* Swift, Jonathan
Wright, Sir Nathan, 22, 83 n. 109, 119

York, John Sharp, Archbishop of, 121